History of The American Academy of Periodontology 1945–1989

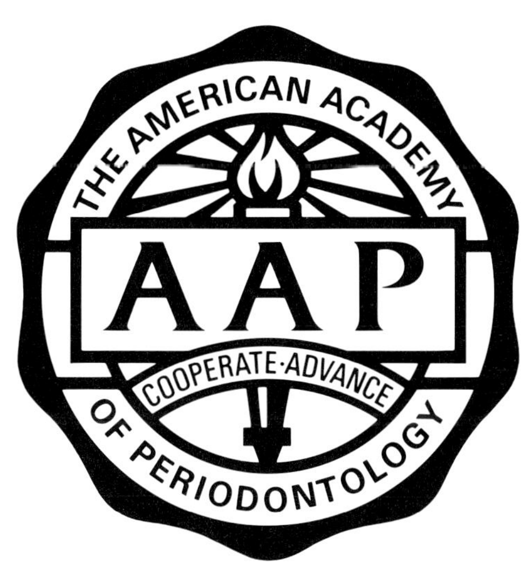

by Maynard K. Hine, D.D.S.

Publication of this history was supported by a grant from W.L. Gore & Associates, Inc. on the occasion of the 75th Anniversary of the American Academy of Periodontology.

TABLE OF CONTENTS

Preface

During the first half of the twentieth century there has been a remarkable growth and development of all facets of dentistry—education, research, techniques, public health, journalism, specialties, and societies. As the public became more aware of the importance of oral health, the demands for dental care increased, and the status of the dental profession improved dramatically.

Prior to this century the attention of most dentists and the public centered around treatment of dental caries, although a few enlightened dentists recognized the importance of periodontology. Excellent histories of the evolution of dentistry, including considerations of periodontal disease have been published and so are not included in this history. Instead, the author concentrated on tracing the development of The American Academy of Periodontology and its influence on periodontology.

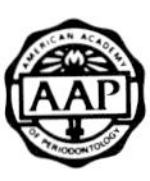

Acknowledgements

Listing the names of those who have assisted in collecting and organizing the text for this book would require considerable space. This text was begun under the aegis of the History Committee and certainly the members of the History Committee should head the list; membership of this committee varied from year to year, but Frank E. Beube, John F. Prichard, Harold Schreiber and B. O. A. Thomas were most active. Marilyn Holmquist assisted in many ways, and Howard Hartman (who serve as the Academy's photographer for many years) supplied many of the photographs included in this book. Perry Ratcliff, Robert Reeves and many others also made significant contributions.

However, as is often true, the chairman must assume the responsibility for the contents of this history. In self defense it must be stated that the collection of data included was time consuming—and frustrating. Some desirable data just could not be located.

It is our hope that this publication will serve as a basis for a future more complete history of the Academy.

Maynard K. Hine, D.D.S.
Chairman
for the History Committee

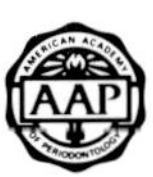

Early Days

In his excellent review of the early years of the American Academy of Periodontology, Dr. Arthur H. Merritt (see Appendix A) wrote that in 1905 Dr. Edward B. Spalding was given permission to invite a group of dentists to spend two or three days in the office of Dr. D. D. Smith of Philadelphia. (Dr. Smith was called by many the "Father of Oral Prophylaxis" as early as 1907). Sixteen of those invited accepted the invitation, and then became enthusiastic supporters of oral prophylaxis. By personal contact, Dr. Smith was able to stimulate interest in a few dentists, but it was the enthusiasm and dedication of Dr. Edward Spalding that gave the field of oral prophylaxis wide publicity.

Dr. Spalding interested a young woman graduate, Dr. Grace Rogers (who later became Mrs. Spalding) to limit her practice to oral prophylaxis. Dr. Merritt gave credit to Dr. Grace Rogers Spalding and another woman, Dr. Gillette Hayden, for the establishment of The American Academy of Periodontology, initially the American Academy of Oral Prophylaxis and Periodontology. There were several dentists who were interested in an organization of periodontists but their proposal was "you women go ahead and organize it, and we'll join." So they did and they did!

There was considerable discussion as to whether the proposed organization should be limited to specialists or be open to general practitioners as well. Some favored a large organization, open to general practitioners. Others wished to limit membership to those practicing periodontics exclusively. Others again suggested two classes of membership—active and associate, one for specialists and one for general practitioners.

From the beginning there were those who were opposed to a separate organization of any kind and those strongly favored the formation of a section in the then National Dental Association (now the American Dental Association) instead. This was especially true of some of the officers and members of that Association. It was also true of several individuals involved in the organization of the Academy. A few, however, held out firmly against such affiliation, notably Drs. Clyde M. Gearhart, Hayden, J. Herbert Hood and Spalding.

It was the original intent of Drs. Hayden and Spalding to create a separate organization and to limit membership to those chiefly interested in the practice of periodontics. It was this plan that was finally adopted.

For the record, an organizing committee met on February 21, 1914, and the an "organization meeting" was held in Cleveland May 23, 1914. Officers, a governing board (called the Council) were elected, and the American Academy of Oral Prophylaxis and Periodontology was underway. Dr. Merritt lists the following individuals who deserve credit for the formation of the Academy:

Gillette Hayden (Columbus, Ohio)
Grace Rogers Spalding (Detroit, Michigan)
John Oppie McCall (Buffalo, New York) [drafted first constitution]
Clyde M. Gearhart (Washington, D.C.)
J. W. Jungman (Cleveland, Ohio)
Austin F. James (Chicago, Illinois)
Andrew J. McDonagh (Toronto, Canada)

The persistence and dedication of these individuals led to the formation of the Academy and provided the basis for its future growth and prosperity. Readers interested in additional information on the early history steady growth of the Academy until 1945 are urged to read the excellent summary by Dr. Merritt.

These pages are designed to present the history of the Academy from 1945 to 1989, which is the seventh-fifth anniversary of its formation.

Brief Overview

In the decade following the end of World War II, periodontology went through a period of very rapid expansion. Funds for research became more readily available, and graduate and postgraduate courses in periodontics multiplied as more and more individuals were attracted to the field of oral health. In 1949 the ADA's House of Delegates recognized the American Board of Periodontology as the official specialty Board for the certification of periodontists. Only one other Board—that of Oral Surgery—had been recognized earlier.

Recognition of periodontology as an official dental specialty increased the interest in periodontics and gave added impetus to its growth. Regulations were established to control the announcements that specialists could make to the public, so certification assumed added importance.

During the 1960s and 1970s developments in periodontology were truly astounding, not only in the scientific aspects of this specialty, but also in its status in the community. Dr. Robert Gottsegen, President of the Academy in 1971, noted in his Presidential Address that there was a "softening of previously fixed positions," and cited "a relaxation of the tight restrictions on what auxiliary personnel, paraprofessionals, are permitted to do, a gradual breaking down of state autonomy in licensure by the formation of Regional Dental Examining Boards, and an about-face on the former total rejection of all prepaid closed-panel systems." There was a growing acceptance of some form of health insurance and, indeed, an eagerness to be included.

In the perspective of the social, economic and cultural changes occurring at every level and in every aspect of dentistry there seemed to be greater responsiveness to public need.

Prevention was being emphasized both in practices and dental school curricula; it became an integral part of being a practitioner and teacher. As Dr. Gottsegen commented, "For periodontists and for the American Academy of Periodontology the focus on prevention is an old story. It has occupied center stage of a large number of our activities for years. Many of our committee members are soldiers grown old in this battle to promote a preventive awareness in the public and a preventive dedication in the profession. Our Public and Professional Relations Committee has made giant strides in these directions. Our Dental Health Plans Committee has been actively engaged in having preventive procedures included as part of the basic package in every dental insurance program. It is vigorously trying, at every opportunity, to make governmental agencies and other third parties accept the concept that treatment of early gingival disease is at least as important as treating early caries. It is struggling to make them accept the fact that there are *two* major dental diseases—not one.

The Academy's success in focusing attention of dental professionals on the periodontal needs of patients did not necessarily carry over into all its efforts to involve the public. Although AAP public relations activities helped to increase public awareness of periodontal disease, some attempts to reach the public directly through action programs and fundraising efforts met with limited success.

During the 1960s, at the instigation of the Committee on Public and Professional

Relations, Citizen Action to Save Teeth (CAST) was formed as a public foundation. It failed to thrive and was discontinued after a few years.

The National Foundation for Prevention of Oral Disease, formed under the leadership of Dr. Perry A. Ratcliff and others in 1971, showed more promise. Its major thrust was first envisioned to be fundraising, but it also promoted public education programs the most successful of which was THETA (Teen Health Education Teaching Assistants). Although the Foundation succeeded in attracting some grants and enough member participation to support a modest central office, it failed to gain significant support from either Academy members, the dental profession, or the public. The Academy, its original sponsor, reluctantly withdrew official sponsorship in 1984 at which time mention of the Foundation was deleted from AAP Bylaws. The Foundation continues to enjoy support of individual AAP members.

In the 1980s increased emphasis was placed on developing educational materials for the public. A committee was appointed to write a brochure on the importance of periodontal recall, to stress the importance of good periodontic root planing, and explain what the recall should include.

In his Presidential Address in 1986, Dr. Robert W. Koch commented that periodontists faced an unusual set of problems and pointed out that the Academy must continue to assume an active leadership role as the authority in periodontics. He said, "This leadership role must be not only with the public, but also within dentistry . . . . Dental products advertising has given us *some* help by making gingivitis a buzzword, but we can't coast on what often are confusing messages to the public . . . . It is our responsibility to provide the public with facts about periodontal disease. We should be willing to help companies provide honest and educational advertising when opportunities are available for this kind of cooperation."

Dr. Koch emphasized that the Academy should continue to intensify its public relations program which "shows every sign of continuing to benefit periodontists and the public." He called attention to the fact that the Academy now had more than 75 committees, and that plans have been developed to set priorities for future goals which will require revising the committee structure.

The Academy has firmly established a leadership role in dentistry, and its leaders have demonstrated the ability and the willingness to meet new challenges as they develop.

Administrative and Governance Structure

Since its organization The American Academy of Periodontology has been fortunate to have dedicated and competent officers and committee chairmen. Most of them were active in the organization for several years before being elected to office; names of many individuals keep recurring as they accepted new responsibilities. During the existence of the American Society of Periodontists (1961–1967) its leaders included many who had been active in the Academy, and they continued to serve after the merger of the two groups.

A full list of Academy Presidents begins on page 82; however, since two of the Secretaries of the Academy served for several years, and they were since responsible for much of the planning and day-to-day management of the Academy until a staffed Central Office was established, it seems appropriate to acknowledge their contributions here.

Dr. Clarke Chamberlain (Peoria, Illinois) was first elected Secretary in 1947 and he served in that capacity until 1964. The AAP Central Office was housed in Dr. Chamberlain's office at 1101 North Street, Peoria, Illinois, until 1965. During those 17 years, the Academy expanded considerably, and the responsibilities of the Secretary grew accordingly. Dr. Chamberlain gradually assumed all the management duties, which required more and more of his time and energy. The Academy owes much to the long and effective service of Dr. Chamberlain.

ESTABLISHMENT OF A CENTRAL OFFICE

When Dr. Chamberlain was elected President-Elect of the Academy in 1965, Dr. Robert Kesel (Aurora, Illinois) assumed the office of Secretary which he held until 1969. Dr. Kesel negotiated a lease for 600 square feet of space in the just completed American Dental Association building at 211 East Chicago Avenue, Chicago, Illinois and on December 1, 1965 the Academy moved in. Dr. Kesel also recruited for the office an assistant with whom he had previously worked on the Survey of Dentistry, Marilyn C. Holmquist. Dr. Kesel had made a commitment to the Academy to spend several mornings a week in the Central Office and provide general oversight, and Ms. Holmquist was to handle administrative details. She was given the title of Assistant Secretary in 1967.

The merger of the Academy and the Society in 1967 and the continual expansion of activities made it clear that additional full time Central Office help was needed. A second staff member was hired in 1967 and in 1968, the Executive Council created the position of Executive Secretary and asked Ms. Holmquist to assume those duties. Additional staff positions have been created over the past 22 years, reflecting AAP's need for expertise in areas such as accounting, meetings management, membership services, public relations, dental prepayment plans, and general association management.

The Executive Secretary, whose title was changed to Executive Director in 1984, retired in December 1986, having completed 21 years of faithful and effective service with the Academy and was succeeded by Alice DeForest.

In his presidential address in 1986, Dr. Robert W. Koch made the following comments about Marilyn Holmquist:

> Marilyn Holmquist will be retiring after twenty-one years with the Academy. No one has dedicated themselves to the good of this Academy and our profession the way Marilyn has. In the time Marilyn has been with the AAP, it has grown from an organization of less that one thousand members to one that is nearly five times that size. She has wrestled with the politics and the personalities and helped keep this organization moving forward. She will leave behind an organization that is energetic and strong, well-staffed and organized. I can't think anything would please her more that knowing she has left us far better than she found us.

As of 1989, the Academy has 23 full time staff positions and office space, still in the ADA building, has grown from the original 600 square feet to nearly 8,000.

GOVERNANCE

The Association is governed by an Executive Council. The Council is composed of the six elected officers (President, President-Elect, Vice President, Secretary, Treasurer, and Immediate Past President) and a total of 21 District members representing seven geographic districts (United States, Puerto Rico, and Canada) and the eighth representing Federal Dental Services. The 21 seats are apportioned on the basis of the number of voting Academy members residing in each district, with each district assured of at least one member. The Council reviews member distribution every three years and reapportions district seats as needed. In addition, the President appoints a non-voting Associate member representative to serve on the Council. The officers are elected by the total voting membership and the district representatives by the voting members in each district.

The Ad Interim Committee serves as the executive body between meetings of the Executive Council and all its actions are subject to ratification by the Council. Its members, as defined in the Bylaws, are the six officers and two district representatives appointed annually by the President.

Appointed Officers

The Bylaws specifically call for two appointed officers, the Executive Director, who administers the facilities and staff for the Academy under the direction of the Council, and the Editor(s) of the *Journal of Periodontology*.

Committees

Because the Academy committee structure is currently undergoing extensive reorganization, it does not seem appropriate to discuss various roles and responsibilities in this publication. Readers interested in this aspect of governance are encouraged to obtain a copy of the Academy's Directory of Members, which includes all the committees and their current membership.

The American Society of Periodontists

During the early years prior to the organization of the American Academy of Periodontology, there was considerable discussion by leading dentists regarding the requirements for admission to membership in an organization to promote periodontology. Some favored including dentists who were *interested* in oral prophylaxis and periodontics, while others wanted the membership limited to those dentists who were teaching or practicing periodontics *exclusively*. Some suggested two classes of membership, "active" for those limiting their practice; "associate" for general practitioners who wanted to learn more about periodontology. The decision was finally made that the Academy should include those "especially interested" in periodontology, but not necessarily limiting their practice to that field.

The debate regarding the importance of an organization controlled by specialists never completely ceased, however. With the development of the American Board of Periodontics in 1939 and the approval of the Board by the American Dental Association in 1948, discussions about the need for having an organization with membership limited to became more intense. Also, the Academy's policy of limiting its membership to 300 active members became a handicap as the numbers of periodontists increased so rapidly.

In 1961 a group of periodontists decided to form the American Society of Periodontists (ASP) with membership restricted to those individuals whose activities were limited to the field of periodontology (Society Bylaws). Membership categories were active, academic, honorary, non-resident and retired. Mr. Morton Stone served as Executive Director for the Society and, following its merger with the Academy, was a member of the AAP staff for several years.

The 1962 Registry of Members of the Society included 240 periodontists from 34 states and Mexico. Interestingly enough practically all Society members were also members of the Academy.

The first Annual Meeting of the Society was held July 5–7, 1962, in Seattle, Washington. It was titled "The Balint Orban Memorial Seminar" and the program included addresses by Drs. Saul Schluger, D. Walter Cohen, Nathan Friedman, Daniel Grant, John Prichard, Clifford Ochsenbein, Henry Goldman, and Harry Bonannan.

The meeting was well attended and it was generally agreed that the Society showed promise of developing into a noteworthy organization.

The Second Annual Meeting of the Society was held on May 5–8, 1963 in Denver, Colorado. A list of the Society's Presidents and can be found on page 90 and the annual meeting sites in Appendix F.

PERIODONTICS, THE JOURNAL OF THE AMERICAN SOCIETY OF PERIODONTISTS

One of the projects of the American Society of Periodontists was to establish a journal. Under the general direction of Dr. Henry M. Goldman, a high–quality scientific publication, *Periodontics* was issued six times a year. A total of six volumes, each of approximately 320 pages were published, from 1963 through 1968. *Periodontics* was well accepted, and helped meet the need for more rapid publication of scientific articles of interest to periodontists.

Dr. Goldman served as Editor and he was assisted by three Associate Editors, Drs. Robert Gottsegen, Daniel Grant, and Timothy J. O'Leary. Dr. John Kollar served as Business Manager and Mr. Morton Stone was Advertising Director.

As explained in the section on publications, *Periodontics* merged with the *Journal of Periodontics* when the two sponsoring organizations united.

Merger of the Society and the Academy

During the 1960s it became generally recognized that it would be in the best interests of periodontists and the public to have one organization represent the area of periodontology to the dental profession, the public, insurance carriers, and the federal government. Many members of both the Academy and the Society spent long hours in the formulation of plans and in exhaustive and exhausting discussions of possible means by which merger might be accomplished. Specific actions were taken by the Academy to attempt to unify the two organizations.

FORMULATION OF A SPECIALIST SECTION OF THE ACADEMY

The first issue of the Academy Newsletter (1966) included the following article, entitled "Uppermost in Our Minds."

> Although a major historical emphasis of the Academy had been the dissemination of periodontal knowledge to the general practitioner, it became apparent several years ago that a sharper focus on the needs of the limited periodontal practitioner was desirable. The Academy therefore undertook to form a Specialist Section. Realizing the implications of such developments as the increased role of the federal government in provision of health services and the advent of dental health insurance, it was hoped that the Specialist Section might also provide a vehicle for merger of the Academy and the Society, whose bylaws restrict Society membership to those who limit their professional activities to the field of periodontology. Because 90% of active Society members are also members of the Academy, merger would do away with the problems of dual membership. To enhance the possibilities of merger, the Academy deferred action on establishment of the Specialist Section for a period of two years (1963–1965) while representatives of both organizations met to consider terms that would be mutually acceptable.
>
> Prior to the 1965 Annual Meeting in Las Vegas, a joint committee composed of Maynard Hine, Donald Kerr, and Charles Williams, representing the Academy, and D. Walter Cohen, William Hiatt, and Saul Schluger, representing the Society, drew up a list of terms for merger that the committee felt would be acceptable to both groups. Because the Specialist Section was to function as the vehicle for merger if and when it was accomplished, this list of terms formed the basis for the amendments drawn up by the Constitution and By-Laws Committee for the purpose of establishing and regulating the Specialist Section. These amendments were sent to all members of the executive bodies of the Academy and the Society so that they could be considered at a meeting of the two bodies on November 1, 1965 in Law Vegas.
>
> The two executive bodies met as scheduled on November 1 to discuss terms of merger. A major item of discussion was the amendments, which

> provided for Section representation on the Executive Council and autonomy in the conduct of Section affairs pertaining to budget and expenditures, election of officers, holding of meetings, and publication of a separate journal. There appeared to be agreement on most of the provisions of the amendments, although some items were left open for further negotiation.
>
> A major point made by the officers of the Society during this meeting was that they felt merger would be unacceptable to the majority of the Society members unless the entire Society membership were accepted for membership in the Section. In deference to this view, at a meeting on November 2 the Executive Council of the Academy unanimously passed a resolution to accept without challenge all active members of the Society for membership in the Section.
>
> At a meeting in April 1966 the joint committee composed of Drs. Cohen, Hiatt, Hine, Kerr, and Williams drew up a list of terms for merger which were presented to the executive body of the Society at its meeting in June 1966 by Dr. Charles Williams. Although no objections were raised, the executive body of the Society declined to take action. The same list of terms was reviewed by the Ad Interim Committee of the Academy at a meeting on August 20, 1966 and was approved unanimously without any change.

Early in 1967, the two executive bodies developed and distributed a questionnaire to all members of both organizations. The results of the questionnaire served as the basis for the deliberations of a joint meeting of the Academy Executive Council and Society Board of Directions in June 1967. Reginald Sullens, then Assistant Secretary of Educational Affairs for the ADA, chaired the two–day session which resulted in a series of recommendations approved by all participants. Among the issues addressed were membership qualifications, committee organization, publication of the respective journals, budget, and governing body structure.

After many conferences and "corridor conversations," a joint meeting of the general assemblies of the Academy and the Society was held during the Academy's 53rd Annual Meeting in Washington, D.C. in October 1967. Nine hundred thirty–five members and guests were on hand to consider the articles of merger and they voted unanimously for approval.

It is tempting to identify by name those individuals who were instrumental in organizing the Society, and those who worked effectively (in public as well as "behind the scenes") for the successful merger. However, the list would vary according to the individual who wrote it. Suffice it to report that all the officers of both organizations were instrumental in preparing and gaining acceptance of a structure which was largely satisfactory to all concerned.

Unbiased individuals agree that the Society focused attention on the need to restructure the Academy, and that the merger resulted in a stronger, more effective organization which benefitted both the memberships and the specialty.

Regional Periodontal Organizations

About the time the Academy and the Society were merging, interest arose in establishing some method of geographic representation on the Academy Executive Council. Because most regions already had periodontal organizations in existence, several of them highly successful and well established, Dr. Perry Ratcliff and others explored with the regional leadership the possibilities of forming a constituent society framework which would be officially linked to AAP.

The result was the formation of the Federation of Regional Organizations, which played an important role in developing the current governance structure of the Academy.

The Federation of Regional Organizations consisted of the following groups: Western Society of Periodontology, Southwest Society of Periodontists, Midwest Society of Periodontology, Southern Academy of Periodontology, Greater Washington Society of Periodontology, Northeastern Society of Periodontists, and Canadian Academy of Periodontology, all of which make significant contributions to the advancement of periodontology.

The Federation did not develop into a constituent society level, mainly due to basic differences in philosophy among the various regional organizations. Some had a long tradition of admitting general dentists as associate members, other strictly limited membership to specialists. Geographic representation was realized in 1974, however, with the creation of eight districts, strictly for the purpose of providing membership on the Executive Council (see Governance Section)

With the implementation of the District system, the Federation was officially disbanded in 1975.

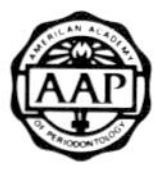

American Board of Periodontology

During the early years of The American Academy of Periodontology there was a growing recognition of the desirability of establishing some qualifications for those who were engaged in the practice of periodontics as a specialty and were announcing that they were indeed specialists.

In his Presidential Report to the Academy in 1937, Dr. Edward Spalding recommended that a committee be appointed to study the specialization concept. As a result of this committee's studies, the American Board of Periodontology was formally organized. The first members of the Board were Drs. Dickson G. Bell of San Francisco; M. Monte Bettman of Portland, Oregon; A. W. Bryan of Iowa City, Iowa (resigned in September 1940); Austin F. James of Chicago, Illinois; Olin Kirkland of Montgomery, Alabama; Harold J. Leonard of New York, New York; and Arthur Merritt of New York, New York. Officers for the year were Dr. Merritt, Chairman; Dr. Kirkland, Vice-Chairman; Dr. Leonard, Secretary-Treasurer.

The Board was incorporated in the State of Illinois in 1940 and approved by the Council on Dental Education of the American Dental Association in 1948.

The primary purposes of the Board were threefold: to set up standards of qualification for those who wish to be recognized as competent periodontists, to examine and certify those who are qualified and wish to be certified, and to publish a roster of those who are certified. A secondary purpose, which is perhaps more important than the primary ones, was to stimulate the development of adequate undergraduate, graduate and post-graduate teaching in periodontology.

Dr. Leonard wrote in an article in the *Journal of Periodontology* that for some time after the organization of the Board, practitioners who had been recognized by their professional conferees as highly efficient in periodontology, had been teaching the subject in dental schools, or had made well-recognized literary and scientific contributions would be certified as diplomates.

The Board is celebrating its 50th anniversary this year and during the past half century, it has certified 837 diplomates (a list of current diplomates can be found in Appendix D).

Over time, the Board has undergone a number of organizational changes, including the number and method of selecting its members, as well as how the examinations are developed and given. Today, there are eight Directors, who must be active members of the Academy and Diplomates of the Board, each of whom serves a single six–year term. Candidates are selected by a Nominating Committee and elected by secret ballot by the voting members of the Academy.

To submit an application for examination by the Board, individuals must hold a degree in dentistry and have successfully completed a study of periodontics in a program accredited by the Commission on Dental Accreditation. The examination consists of three parts, which must be taken in the following sequence: a written examination given annually, case report screening, and a case report/oral examination. Following successful completion of the written exam, a candidate is granted a six–year period during which the remainder of the examination process must be completed.

The Board has been a very important force in upgrading periodontology as a specialty and much credit should be given to the Directors. They have all been dedicated, serious, and much credit should be given to the Directors. They have all been dedicated, serious, and competent individuals who have devoted a great amount of time and energy to the vital, but often thankless, job of establishing and maintaining the high standards requirement for recognition as a Diplomate.

DIRECTORS OF THE AMERICAN BOARD OF PERIODONTOLOGY

Harold J. Leonard, 1940–1958
Arthur H. Merritt, 1940–1955
Dickson G. Bell, 1940–1951
M. Monte Bettman, 1940–1954
Olin Kirkland, 1940–1947
Austin F. James, 1940–1947
A. W. Bryan, 1940
Edgar D. Coolidge, 1940–1942
Bernard Friedman, 1940–1942
Clarke E. Chamberlain, 1947–1964
Samuel R. Parks, 1947–1954
Raymond E. Johnson, 1951–1960
Harry Lyons, 1955–1961
Henry Goldman, 1954–1959
B.O.A. Thomas, 1954–1960
Maynard K. Hine, 1958–1962
Donald Kerr, 1959–1965
Harold G. Ray, 1959–1960
John W. Neilson, 1960–1966
Frank E. Beube, 1960–1968
Henry W. Swenson, 1962–1970
Erwin M. Schaffer, 1964–1970
Claude L. Nabers, 1965–1971
Robert L. Reeves, 1966–1971
D. Walter Cohen, 1966–1972
Sigurd P. Ramfjord, 1968–1974
Timothy O'Leary, 1970–1976
John F. Prichard, 1970–1976
S. Sigmund Stahl, 1971–1977
Saul Schluger, 1972–1978
Gerald M. Kramer, 1972–1978
Robert G. Schallhorn, 1974–1980
Gerald M. Bowers, 1976–1983
Leonard Hirschfeld, 1976–1981
Clifford Ochsenbein, 1976–1982
Billy Pennel, 1977–1979
Herman Corn, 1977–1983
Sheldon D. Benjamin, 1978–1981
Richard Chace, 1978–1984
John Prichard, 1979–1980
R. Earl Robinson, 1980–1985
Abram I. Chasens, 1980–1986
Daniel A. Grant, 1981–1987
Anthony Gargiulo, 1982–1988
Robert Gottsegen, 1982–1988
Philip Hoag, 1983–1989
William Becker, 1983–1989
Walter Donnenfeld, 1984–1990
Dan Loughlin, 1985–1991
Erwin Barrington, 1986–1992
Raymond Yukna, 1987–1993
Jack Caton, 1988–1994
James Mellonig, 1988–1994

Publications

JOURNAL OF PERIODONTOLOGY

The *Journal of Periodontology* has long been one of the outstanding contributions of the American Academy of Periodontology to the development of periodontics. The first Academy president, Dr. Austin James, recognized the importance of such a publication, and recommended in his presidential address in 1915 that one be established. However, the first issue of the *Journal* did not appear until January 1930. The death of Dr. Gillette Hayden in 1929, a stauch supporter of the Academy and of periodontology, motivated the Committee on Dental Educational Bulletins to establish a periodical to be dedicated to her and her many contributions.

The first issue of the *Journal*, which was edited by the Academy's Committee on Dental Educational Bulletins with Harold J. Leonard chairman, consisted of 26 pages devoted to the program of the 16th Annual Meeting of the Academy, reports of committees, memorial resolutions, and the preliminary program for the 17th Annual Meeting. The second number of Volume 1 was also scheduled for publication in 1930, but sufficient material was not available, so the second issue was published in January, 1931.

During the early years, Dr. Grace Rogers Spalding worked actively for the *Journal*, although she was listed as only a member of the committee responsible for the Academy's publications. Dr. Spalding was identified as Editor in 1933, and served in that post until July 1950, with Drs. Harold J. Leonard and Arthur Merritt as associate editors. During this period, the *Journal* expanded into a solid scientific publication and began appearing quarterly in 1946. When Dr. Spalding decided that she could no longer continue her responsibilities, the Executive Council appointed Dr. Maynard K. Hine Editor and named Dr. Spalding as Editor Emeritus. For the next 15 years Dr. Hine and his office staff were almost solely responsible for the many editorial and bookkeeping duties required in the production of a scientific journal. During this time the circulation multiplied six–fold and the size of the *Journal* increased year by year. In 1965, the growing realization that other assignments were interfering with the publication of this modern scientific specialty journal, caused the Editor to search for help, and fortunately he was able to convince Dr. Timothy J. O'Leary to serve as his assistant.

During the early years, the *Journal* accepted no advertising, but as costs of publication increased, the Executive Council finally authorized acceptance of advertisements beginning with the January–February 1966 issue. There was some criticism of this action, particularly by older members, but since the only ads accepted were for products of interest to periodontists and which had been approved by the appropriate ADA Council, the criticism soon dissipated. The Guidelines for appropriate advertising have been revised over the years and acceptance is now determined by a Screening Committee.

As noted earlier, the American Society of Periodontists sponsored an excellent publication, *Periodontics*, with Dr. Henry M. Goldman as its first (and only) editor. With the merger of the *Journal of Periodontology* with *Periodontics* in 1969, Dr. Hine agreed to serve as coordinator for a transition period, during which Dr. Goldman and Dr. O'Leary were actually responsible for the details of publication. In 1969, the publication carried both titles, but it was mutually agreed that future issues should be known as the *Journal of Periodontology*. The *Journal* became a monthly publication with the January 1969 issue.

In 1970 Dr. Hine resigned and was named Editor Emeritus and Dr. Goldman and Dr. O'Leary were appointed Co-Editors. In 1980 Dr. Goldman found it necessary to resign, and so joined Dr. Hine as Editor Emeritus. Dr. William C. Hurt was appointed Co-Editor with Dr. O'Leary and these two assumed responsibilities for alternate issues of the *Journal*, assisted by a group of 25 to 30 "consultants" who reviewed articles for publication.

Drs. O'Leary and Hurt resigned in 1988 and were succeeded by Dr. Robert J. Genco, who thus became the sixth Editor of the *Journal of Periodontology* which will enter its seventh decade of publication in January 1990.

This brief history of the *Journal of Periodontology* indicates that in the first 20 years of publication, the *Journal* became well established; in the second 20 years it developed to an internationally respected specialty journal; and the *Journal* has continued to expand in every way. In 1988, the *Journal* contained 870 pages and about 100 pages of ads. It is a well-recognized scientific journal and is widely cited. Truly the Academy can be proud of the *Journal of Periodontology*.

OTHER PUBLICATIONS

The Academy also issues many other publications designed to inform its members and sometimes the public of recent developments related to periodontics. The ones mentioned below are representative of those now available.

The *AAP News* is a bimonthly newsletter which features a President's message, information about AAP Annual Meetings, upcoming and important national and international events, occasionally summaries of important symposia, practices for sale, academic opportunities, etc. The *News* is sent to all Academy members, dental libraries, and others.

The Constitution and Bylaws of the Academy is published annually in the *Directory of Members*. Reflecting the dynamic nature of the organization, it is revised on an annual basis. The most current document is included as Appendix B.

The *Directory of Members* is distributed annually to all members and includes, in additional to alphabetical and geographic membership lists, much pertinent information about the Academy such as Committee members, Constitution and Bylaws, Past Presidents, Honorary Members, Fellows, Diplomates of the American Board, and descriptions of all available publications.

Professional and educational materials include proceedings from three Workshops sponsored by the Academy in 1966, 1977, and 1989; *Current Procedural Terminology for Periodontics; Glossary of Periodontic Terms;* and a variety of patient education materials.

Honors and Awards

The American Academy of Periodontology annually recognizes several individuals for their contributions to the art and science of periodontology in many ways. Following is a summary of the Academy awards.

GOLD MEDAL AWARD

This award, which is given annually in recognition of outstanding contributions to the field of periodontics, was established by the American Society of Periodontists in 1967, and since merger, by the Academy.

Recipients

1967, Sumter Arnim
1968, Henry M. Goldman
1969, Maynard K. Hine
1970, Harry Sicher
1971, D. Walter Cohen
1972, Irving Glickman*
1973, Sigurd P. Ramfjord
1974, John F. Prichard
1975, Saul Schluger
1976, Balint Orban*
1977, Timothy J. O'Leary
1978, Claude L. Nabers
1979, Jens Waerhaug
1980, Helmut Zander
1981, Robert L. Reeves
1982, S. Sigmund Stahl
1983, Clifford Ochsenbein
1984, Charles W. Finley
1985, Henry M. Swenson
1986, Abram I. Chasens
1987, Marvin Sugarman
1988, Robert Gottsegen
1989, Robert G. Schallhorn

*awarded posthumously

THE WILLIAM J. GIES AWARD IN PERIODONTOLOGY

The William J. Gies Award in Periodontology in memory of Arthur Hastings Merritt was established in 1964 by the William J. Gies Foundation for the Advancement of Dentistry in collaboration with the American Academy of Periodontology, and recognizes outstanding contributions in the field of periodontology. The occasion was the fiftieth anniversary meeting of the Academy.

The award was established to honor Dr. William John Gies, a noted biochemist, and Dr. Arthur Hastings Merritt, famous periodontist and an active Academy member. These gentlemen were close personal friends who set such high standards of achievement in advancing dental health service and in promoting the best in professional ideals and they set a goal for all to strive for.

The plaque consists of an etching of the cover of the March 1876 issue of the *Pennsylvania Journal of Dental Science* which included the memorable paper by John Riggs on "Suppurative Inflammation of the Gums and Absorption of the Gums and Alveolar Process." The portrait of Dr. John Riggs overlays the etching and serves as a reminder that his classic description and recommended therapy of periodontal disease stands as valid today as it did that day when he first penned it almost a century ago. Candidates for the award are submitted by the Academy with the recipient selected by the Foundation.

Recipients

1964, Edgar D. Coolidge
1965, Harry Lyons
1966, Harold J. Leonard
1967, Maynard K. Hine
1968, John Oppie McCall
1969, Joseph L. Bernier
1970, Irving Glickman and Henry M. Goldman
1971, Sigurd Ramfjord
1972, Timothy J. O'Leary
1973, Perry A. Ratcliff
1974, Erwin M. Schaffer
1975, D. Walter Cohen
1976, S. Sigmund Stahl
1977, John F. Prichard
1978, Harold Löe
1979, Frank E. Beube
1980, Paul N. Baer
1981, Max Listgarten
1982, Roy C. Page
1983, Robert J. Genco
1984, Gerald M. Bowers
1985, Helmut Zander
1986, Sigmund S. Socransky
1987, Gerald M. Bowers
1988, Sebastian Ciancio
1989, Raul G. Caffessee

HONORARY MEMBERSHIP

A person who has made outstanding contributions to the art and science of periodontology may be classified as an Honorary Member. He/she may or may not be a member of the Academy at the time the honor is given. Election is by the General Assembly. A certificate of Honorary membership is sent to the candidate(s) following election to this category of membership. Since this recognition is a membership category, only currently living Honorary members are listed below.

Recipients

Ernest H. Besch, 1979
Lester W. Burket*
John M. Coady, 1984
Maynard K. Hine, 1970
Marilyn C. Holmquist, 1973
Gerald H. Leatherman
Thomas Lehner, 1979
Jan L. Lindhe, 1982
Irwin D. Mandel, 1975
A.H. Melcher*
Hans R. Muhlemann, 1981
E. Jean Pierson, 1983
Robert W. Rule, Jr.*
Sigmund S. Socransky, 1984
Morton B. Stone, 1975
Helmut A. Zander, 1972

*date not available.

FELLOWSHIPS

Fellows of the Academy are chosen for distinguished service to the Academy, and election is by the Executive Council. A Certificate of Fellowship is presented to the member(s) so honored.

Recipients

James E. Aiguier, 1962
Stanley C. Baker*
Erwin P. Barrington, 1982
Frank E. Beube, 1978
B. Charles Bruce, 1986
Richard Chace, 1985
Abram I. Chasens, 1982
Sebastian Ciancio, 1987
D. Walter Cohen, 1977
Herman Corn, 1984
Frank G. Everett, 1975
Charles W. Finley, 1983
Irving Glickman, 1971
Henry M. Goldman*
Stephen F. Goodman, 1988
Robert Gottsegen, 1981
Howard Hartman, 1972
William H. Hiatt, 1985
Maynard K. Hine
Leonard Hirschfeld, 1988
William C. Hurt, 1984
Raymond E. Johnson*
Donald A. Kerr*
Robert G. Kesel, 1962
Robert Koch, 1989
Kenneth Langley, 1989
Walter Leabo*
Harold J. Leonard*
Max Listgarten, 1988
Harry Lyons, 1958
Joseph E. Maybury, 1987
John Oppie McCall*
Russell A. McCallion, 1987
Harold L. Meador, 1979
Claude L. Nabers, 1976
James Y. O'Bannon, 1979
Timothy J. O'Leary, 1975
Roy C. Page, 1989
John S. Pfeifer, 1986
John F. Prichard, 1971
Sigurd P. Ramfjord, 1981
Robert L. Reeves, 1978
Perry A. Ratcliff*
Erwin M. Schaffer, 1977
Saul Schluger, 1972
S. Sigmund Stahl, 1983
Marvin M. Sugarman, 1980
Henry M. Swenson, 1976
B. O. A. Thomas*
James A. Tobias, 1980
Charles H.M. Williams, 1970
Helmut Zander, 1974

*date not available

SPECIAL CITATIONS

The Executive Council can authorize the awarding of special citations to individuals who have contributed to the work of the Academy in a noteworthy manner, specifically in committee service or a special project.

Recipients

Arnold A. Ariaudo, 1975
Erwin P. Barrington, 1979
Gerald M. Bowers, 1982
B. Charles Bruce, 1984
Sebastian Ciancio, 1983
H. Dalton Conner, 1988
Chester Douglass, 1986
Gordon L. Douglass, 1989
Robert T. Ferris, 1987
Charles W. Finley, 1976
William B. Gillette, 1989
Stephen F. Goodman, 1984
J. Richard Hall, 1984
Marilyn C. Holmquist, 1985
Bennett Klavan, 1981
Merwyn A. Landay, 1975
Milton A. Marten, 1987
Donald H. Masters, 1975
Russell A. McCallion, 1986
Harold L. Meador, 1975
James Mellonig, 1988
Myron Nevins, 1980
E. Jean Pierson, 1980
David Plessett, 1988
Morton B. Stone, 1981
Leonard S. Tibbetts, 1987
James A. Tobias, 1977
Ronald Von Swol, 1987
Richard D. Wilson, 1989
Raymond Yukna, 1988

BALINT ORBAN MEMORIAL PROGRAM

The Orban Competition was begun by the American Society of Periodontists. When the AAP/ASP merger took place in 1967, the Academy agreed to fulfill the meeting commitments of the Society so there were spring as well as fall meetings in 1968 and 1969 and a Balint Orban Prize Competition at both. At the June 1968 and the October 1969 meetings there was also a Graduate Student Seminar. In 1970 these two programs were given jointly as the Graduate Student Program and the Balint Orban Prize Competition.

The rules were rewritten in 1970 combining the two programs formally under the name Balint Orban Memorial Program and these were approved by the Executive Council.

Recipients

Robert L. Burns, 1968
Russell J. Nisengard
and Richard R. Ranney, 1969
Steven E. Berglund, 1970
Leonard Shapiro, 1971
Robert E. Lamb, 1972
Robert D. Kiger, 1973
David Movius, 1974
Michael G. Newman, 1975
Mark R. Patters, 1976
Dennis H. Smith, 1977
Eugene T. Altiere, 1978
Jane M. Jensen, 1979
Jeffrey Gordon, 1980
Thomas E. Van Dyke, 1981
Jon B. Suzuki, 1982
John E. Duckwork, 1983
Michael P. Rethman, 1984
Philip J. Hanes, 1985
Charlene B. Krejci, 1986
Francis G. Serio, 1987
Bryan S. Michalorwicz, 1988

PRESIDENTIAL AWARD

Established in 1987, the recipient is elected by the Executive Council and presented to an Academy member for distinguished service to the Academy over a period of years.

Recipients

1987, Maynard K. Hine
1988, Frank Beube
1989, William C. Hurt

MASTER CLINICIAN AWARD

Also established in 1987, this award is presented to an Academy member who has practiced and demonstrated consistent clinical excellence in periodontics and who has willingly and unselfishly shared this clinical expertise with members of the profession.

Recipients

1987, Herman Corn
1988, John F. Prichard
1989, Gerald M. Kramer

CLINICAL RESEARCH AWARD

This annual award honors the most outstanding scientific manuscript which has direct clinical relevance and application to the practice of periodontics and which has been published in the refereed scientific literature within the prior calendar year. The Committee on Research in Periodontology nominates the manuscripts and final selection is made by the Executive Council.

Recipients

1984 Alan M. Polson. "Effect of Periodontal Trauma on Intrabony Pockets" *J Periodontol* 54:586, 1983.

1985 William Becker. "Periodontal Treatment Without Maintenance: A Retrospective Study in 44 Patients" *J Periodontol* 55:505, 1984.

1986 James E. Kennedy, William C. Bird, Kent G. Palcanis, and Howard S. Dorfman. "A Longitudinal Evaluation of Varying Width of Attached Gingiva" *J Clin Periodontol 12*:667, 1985.

1987 M.A. Listgarten, C.C. Schifter, P. Sullivan, C. George, and E.S. Rosenberg. "Failure of a Microbial Assay to Reliably Predict Disease Recurrence in a Treated Periodontist Population Receiving Regularly Scheduled Prophylaxis" *J Clin Periodontol 13*:768–773, 1986.

1988 B.L. Pihlstrom, L.F. Wolff, M.B. Bakdash, E.M. Schaffer. J.R. Jensen, Jr., D.A. Aeppli, and O.L. Bandt. "Salt and Peroxide Compared With Conventional Oral Hygiene—I. Clinical Results." *J Periodont. 58*:291–300, 1987.
L.F. Wolff, B.L. Pihlstrom, M.B. Bakdash, E.M. Schaffer, J.R. Jensen Jr., D.M. Aeppli, and C.L. Bandt. "Salt and Peroxide Compared With Conventional Oral Hygiene—II. Microbial Results." *J Periodontol 58*:301–307, 1987.

M.B. Bakdash, L.F. Wolff, B.L. Pihlstrom, D.M. Aeppli, and C.L. Bandt. "Salt and Peroxide Compared With Conventional Oral Hygiene—III. Patient Compliance And Acceptance" *J Periodontol 58*:308–313, 1987.

1989 W. Becker, B.E. Becker, C. Ochsenbein, G. Kerry, R. Caffesse, E.C. Morrison, and J. Prichard. "A Longitudinal Study Comparing Scaling, Osseous Surgery And Modified Widman Procedures. Results After One Year" *J Periodontol 59*:351–365, 1988.

R. EARL ROBINSON PERIODONTAL REGENERATION AWARD

This award will first be given at the 1989 Annual Meeting and was established by Dr. Robinson to encourage research in periodontal regeneration by recognizing the author(s) of the peer–reviewed paper which has contributed most to the knowledge of periodontal regeneration during the previous calendar year.

Recipients

Schallhorn, R.G. and McClain, P.K. "Combined Osseous Composite Grafting, Root Conditioning, and Guided Tissue Regeneration." *Intern J Periodontics Restorative Dent* 8(1):9–31, 1988.

Appendix A

HISTORY OF THE AMERICAN ACADEMY OF PERIODONTOLOGY

By ARTHUR H. MERRITT, D.D.S., F.A.A.P.

Preface

AT A MEETING of the Executive Council of the American Academy of Periodontology on February 22, 1943, a suggestion was made by Dr. Samuel R. Parks, then President-elect, that a history of the organization and early activities of the society be written while a few of those responsible were yet living. It was first thought that this could best be done by one of the organizers, and all signs pointed to Dr. Grace Rogers Spalding as the logical author. She had been one of the Founders of the Academy and had played a conspicuous part in its organization and subsequent progress. Probably no one had so intimate a knowledge of its history as she. But she promptly pointed out that since she had been active in its organization, she could not for that reason undertake the writing of its history. At a later conference on the subject, in May, 1945, it became increasingly evident that if a history of the Academy was to be written, it would need to be done by some one who had had no part in its organization and who could therefore write objectively without the embarrassment of having been an active participant in its early development. Since the author met these requirements and was fully familiar with Academy traditions—having been a member for nearly thirty years—he was asked to write this history. And so, when Dr. Spalding generously offered to place at his disposal such data as she had in her possession, what else could he do but accept? Which is the author's only excuse for having undertaken the task.

A.H.M.

Note: Original Citation: *J Periodontol.* 1947; 18:121–142.

Introduction

THROUGHOUT recorded history there have been two major disorders which have brought about the loss of teeth. One, known as caries, was obvious, painful, and destructive. It was also one which could be somewhat controlled by the application of mechanical measures. The second, involving the periodontal tissues and known by a multitude of names, was more subtle and in its early stages more or less painless. It called for quite a different type of treatment of which there was little knowledge, and one in which mechanical procedures played a relatively small part.

When dentistry as an organized profession came into being in this country (and throughout the century which has since elapsed,) its attention was largely directed toward the repair and replacement of teeth affected by caries. That it should have done so is easily understood. Caries made its appearance early in life. It was painful and disfiguring. Unless controlled, many teeth—probably most of them—would be lost in childhood and adolescence. To meet this situation, American dentistry focused attention largely upon the control of dental caries by the exercise of technical procedures of one kind or another. In so doing it has achieved a perfection in these procedures which has made the name of American dentistry the synonym for excellence throughout the civilized world.

Meanwhile, relatively little consideration had been given to that other group of diseases which affect and tend to destroy the periodontal tissues. One of the results has been that periodontoclasia, one of this group of diseases, is at present responsible for the loss of more teeth than any other disease.[1] It was out of deep concern for this situation, and with a view to remedying it, that the American Academy of Periodontology came into being.

1 Brekus, P. J., A Report on Loss of Teeth. *J.A.D.A.* Vol. 25, p: 679

I

Pioneers In Periodontia

HERE AND THERE throughout the country there were members of the dental profession who came to realize the importance of oral hygiene and to emphasize its value as a preventive measure. Among its early advocates were those whose attention was still focused on dental caries—hence the slogan, "Clean teeth do not decay". There were others, however, who recognized the wider implications of oral prophylaxis (as the means used to promote oral hygiene came to be known) namely, its importance in the prevention and treatment of periodontal disorders.

Among these was Dr. Levi C. Taylor of Hartford, Conn. Beginning in 1868, Dr. Taylor spent two years in the office of Dr. John M. Riggs where he got his first impressions of the importance of oral prophylaxis by noting the failure of proper postoperative care. "Dr. Riggs" he said "would treat a case better the first time even, than any man I ever knew, but as soon as completed he would remark, 'Come in again in a little while and we will go over them again'. This meant nothing until the mouth was nearly as bad as before." (Letter to E.B.S. June 9, 1906.)

One of the later crusaders in the field of oral prophylaxis was Dr. Alfred C. Fones (1869-1938) of Bridgeport, Conn. So impressed was he with the importance of regular prophylactic care, he founded the first school for the teaching of young women to give such treatments,—an innovation which has taken its place in dental practice despite some opposition. Apropos of the experiment Dr. Levi Taylor makes this observation: "Dr. Fones does fine work personally but his theory of the Dental Nurse will *never do.*"

Foremost among the early promoters of oral prophylaxis was Dr. D. D. Smith (1839-1920) of Philadelphia who as early as 1907 was referred to as the "Father of Oral Prophylaxis".[2] Beginning in the latter part of the 19th century, and continuing up to the time of his death in 1920, Smith published many articles on the general subject of oral prophylaxis. (The titles of twenty are before me as I write.) This he defined as the "careful and complete removal of all calcic deposits, inspissated secretions, bacterial plaques and all accretions that gather on the surfaces of the teeth and between them, especially at the gum margins, followed by thorough polishing of all tooth surfaces by hand methods". The results which he obtained were reported as remarkable. A few, interested in the work he was doing made pilgrimages to his office and came away thoroughly convinced of the importance of oral prophylaxis in the practice of dentistry.

2 *Dental Summary*, Vol. 27, p. 561.

One of these was Dr. Edward B. Spalding of Detroit, who for several years had been interested in oral prophylaxis, writing two papers on the subject in 1905. Greatly impressed with what he saw in Dr. Smith's office, he was given permission to invite a number of dentists to spend two or three days in Smith's office in April 1906, to see for themselves the extraordinary results accomplished by regular prophylactic care. Sixteen of those invited accepted the invitation—one of this number last served on the Organization Committee and four were among the earliest members of the Academy. They came, they saw for themselves, and returned to their offices enthusiastic supporters of oral prophylaxis. "We were prepared" one of those present reported, "to see good results, but we were greatly surprised to see such a uniform lot of perfectly healthy and clean mouths, most of which had been redeemed from what had evidently been desperate cases of pyorrhea".[3]

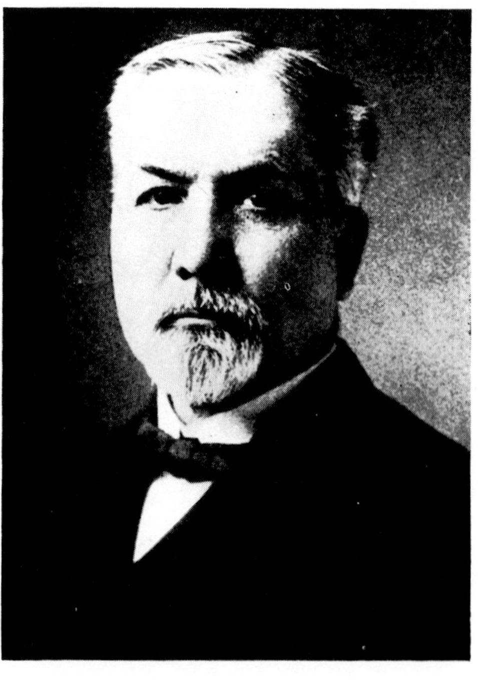

D. D. SMITH, M.D., D.D.S.

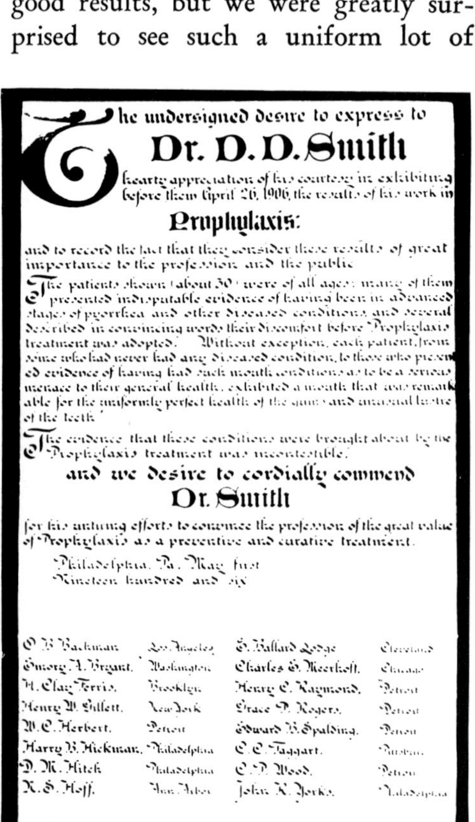

The undersigned desire to express to

Dr. D. D. Smith

hearty appreciation of his courtesy in exhibiting before them April 26, 1906, the results of his work in

Prophylaxis:

and to record the fact that they consider these results of great importance to the profession and the public.

The patients shown (about 30) were of all ages; many of them presented indisputable evidence of having been in advanced stages of pyorrhea and other diseased conditions, and several described in convincing words their discomfort before Prophylaxis treatment was adopted. Without exception, each patient, from some who had never had any diseased condition, to those who presented evidence of having had such mouth conditions as to be a serious menace to their general health, exhibited a mouth that was remarkable for the uniformly perfect health of the gums and natural lustre of the teeth.

The evidence that these conditions were brought about by the Prophylaxis treatment was incontestible.

and we desire to cordially commend

Dr. Smith

for his untiring efforts to convince the profession of the great value of Prophylaxis as a preventive and curative treatment.

Philadelphia, Pa., May first
Nineteen hundred and six

O. B. Backman	Los Angeles	S. Ballard Lodge	Cleveland
Emory A. Bryant.	Washington	Charles S. Meerhoff.	Chicago
H. Clay Ferris.	Brooklyn	Henry C. Raymond.	Detroit
Henry W. Gillett.	New York	Grace P. Rogers.	Detroit
W. C. Herbert.	Detroit	Edward B. Spalding.	Detroit
Harry B. Hickman.	Philadelphia	C. C. Taggart.	[illegible]
D. M. Hitch	Philadelphia	C. P. Wood.	Detroit
R. S. Hoff.	Ann Arbor	John R. Yorks.	Philadelphia

Dr. D. D. Smith was an exceptionally skillful dentist. His crown and bridgework was remarkably well executed, but because of what seems to have been a somewhat autocratic nature, Dr. Smith was never highly successful in getting his message of Oral Prophylaxis over to the profession. He was by nature, arbitrary, dogmatic, and unapproachable. Credit for appreciating the value of Smith's work in this field and for giving it wide publicity belongs largely to Dr. Edward B. Spalding. It was he who was instrumental in introducing oral prophylaxis into Europe through his acquaintance with Drs. Robert McBride and N. S. Jenkins of Dresden. Believing that women dentists were especially adapted for this type of practice, Dr. Spalding in 1904 persuaded Dr. Grace Rogers, a young graduate, to spend a year in postgraduate work at the University of Michigan in preparation for limiting her practice to oral prophylaxis in 1905. Through their united influence, in 1906 Drs. McBride and Jenkins engaged Dr. Gillette Hayden of Columbus, Ohio, to take up its practice in their office in Dresden, Germany, where she remained for three years. She was asked by them to visit the offices of Drs. Smith and Spalding before sailing for Europe. It was Dr. Spalding's enthusiasm, plus that of his associate, which was a definite influence in setting in motion the forces which culminated in the birth of the American Academy of Periodontology. The majority of the charter members were followers of Dr. D. D. Smith.

II

First Steps In Organization

THE IDEA of an organization for the promotion of oral prophylaxis and all it implied, was a natural outgrowth of the interest created by such men as Dr. D. D. Smith and his small group of followers.

A careful study of correspondence and official records of what took place in those early days, clearly points to the fact that the vision of an organization such as has come to be known as the American Academy of Periodontology, had its birth in the minds of two women—Drs. Gillette Hayden and Grace Rogers Spalding. It is not too much to say that but for their enthusiasm and perseverance, plus the encouragement received from Drs. James, Spalding, McCall and others consulted, an organization in periodontia would not have come into being when it did. To them, more than to any others belongs the credit for visioning the possibilities of such an organization and for the high ideals which have always characterized it. During 1913 and early 1914, these two women came together several times to discuss ways and means for translating their vision into a reality.

While at the meeting of the National Dental Association at Kansas City in 1913, Drs. Hayden and Spalding approached Dr. John D. Patterson of that city and Dr. J. W. Jungman of Cleveland regarding their plan. Their only comment was "You women go ahead and organize it and we'll join".

Following the meeting of the Ohio State Dental Society at Toledo in December 1913, Dr. Spalding returned to Columbus with Dr. Hayden for the purpose of making definite plans for the formation of an organization such as they had had under consideration for a year or more. Having arrived at the decision to put the plan into effect following a further conference in Detroit in January, 1914, steps were taken to bring together the Organization Committee, Dr. Hayden meanwhile acting as chairman and Dr. Spalding as secretary. The following agreed to serve on the Committee: A. C. Hamm of Denver, Clyde M. Gearhart of Washington, John O. McCall of Buffalo, and J. W. Jungman of Cleveland. Dr. T. Sydney Smith of San Francisco was asked to join the Committee but was unable to do so. The Committee was invited to Cleveland. Of those invited, all except Drs. Smith, Hamm and Gearhart accepted the invitation and met in Dr. Jungman's office on February 21, 1914 with Dr. J. Herbert Hood substituting for Dr. Smith, making five in all—Drs. Hayden, Spalding, McCall, Jungman and Hood.

Considerable discussion developed as to whether the proposed organization should be limited to specialists or be open to general practitioners. Some favored a large organization, open to general practitioners. Others wished to limit membership to those practicing periodontia exclusively. Others again suggested two classes of membership—active and associate.

From the beginning there had been those who were opposed to a *separate organization* of any kind and who strongly favored the formation of a section in the then National Dental Association, instead. This was especially true of some of the officers and members of that Association. It was also true of several having to do with the organization of the Academy. A few, however, held out firmly against such affiliation, notably Drs. Gearhart, Hayden, Hood, and Spalding.

It had all along been the purpose of Drs. Hayden and Spalding to create a separate organization and to limit membership to those chiefly interested in the practice of periodontia. It was this plan that was finally adopted. In the Preamble (dated February 21, 1914), setting forth its objectives, the statement is made that, "We, the undersigned, do hereby deem it for the best interests of the public and the profession that a society should be formed to the end that those especially interested may meet and work together without prejudice for the scientific investigation of caries and periodontoclasia; that the practice of Oral Prophylaxis and Periodontia as an exclusive specialty may be encouraged . . ." Signed:

Grace Rogers Spalding	J. H. Hood
Gillette Hayden	A. C. Hamm
C. M. Gearhart	J. O. McCall
J. W. Jungman	

A preliminary draft of a constitution and by-laws prepared by Dr. John O. McCall was submitted for consideration at this time. Each member of the Committee was requested to submit the names of those who might be eligible to membership. From this list were chosen the names of those who were later invited to attend the Organization Meeting. The Committee then adjourned to meet again in Cleveland, May 23, 1914.

III

Organization Meeting

THE Organization Committee having decided to form a society for promoting the study and practice of periodontology, the group which came together in Cleveland May 23, 1914, had as its purpose the formation of such a society. The following were designated as Charter Members:

DR. GILLETTE HAYDEN, *Columbus, Ohio*
DR. GRACE ROGERS SPALDING, *Detroit, Michigan*
DR. CLYDE M. GEARHART, *Washington, D. C.*
DR. JOHN O. MCCALL, *Buffalo, N. Y.*
DR. J. W. JUNGMAN, *Cleveland, Ohio*
DR. A. C. HAMM, *Denver, Colo.*
DR. J. HERBERT HOOD, *Cleveland, Ohio*
DR. AUSTIN F. JAMES, *Chicago, Ill.*
DR. ANDREW J. MCDONAGH, *Toronto, Can.*
DR. MARY E. ALLEYNE, *Detroit, Mich.*
DR. CHARLES P. WOOD, *Detroit, Mich.*
DR. R. R. JOHNSTON, *Pittsburgh, Pa.*
DR. L. D. CORIELL, *Baltimore, Md.*
DR. EDNA WITBECK NOYES, *Detroit, Mich.*
DR. R. G. HUTCHINSON, JR., *New York City*
DR. E. GRACE KEITH, *Portland, Oregon*
DR. ALICE HARVEY DUDEN, *Indianapolis, Ind.*
DR. M. LOUISE PAGELSEN, *Detroit, Mich.*

(It will be noted that of the eighteen charter members more than one third were women, and all but three were by that time limiting their practices to oral prophylaxis and periodontia.)

From those present the following officers were elected:

President, AUSTIN F. JAMES, *Chicago*
First Vice-President, ANDREW J. MCDONAGH, *Toronto*
Second Vice-President, R. G. HUTCHINSON, JR., *New York City*
Secretary, CHARLES P. WOOD, *Detroit*
Treasurer, MARY E. ALLEYNE, *Detroit*

The election of a governing board (called the Council) completed the organization. Drs. Hayden, Spalding, James, McCall, Gearhart, McDonagh, Jungman, and Hood were among the most active at the Organization Meeting. All were in dead earnest. To Drs. Hayden and Spalding it was a matter of life and death. Their long cherished dream had finally become a reality. To them should be given the credit for conceiving the idea and for their perseverance in bringing it to fruition. Dr. John O. McCall submitted for consideration a revised draft of the Constitution and By-laws which was "adopted and subscribed to by 18 charter members, 10 of whom were present". (Gillette Hayden's presidential address—1915.)

After discussion of other organizational matters, the meeting adjourned to meet at Rochester, N. Y., July 10, 1914. This was a brief business session somewhat in the nature of a second organization meeting. The constitution and by-laws, the question of dues, and the choice of the next meeting place were the chief topics for discussion. Having voted to hold its first annual meeting in Washington, D. C., in November 1914, the Rochester session was adjourned.

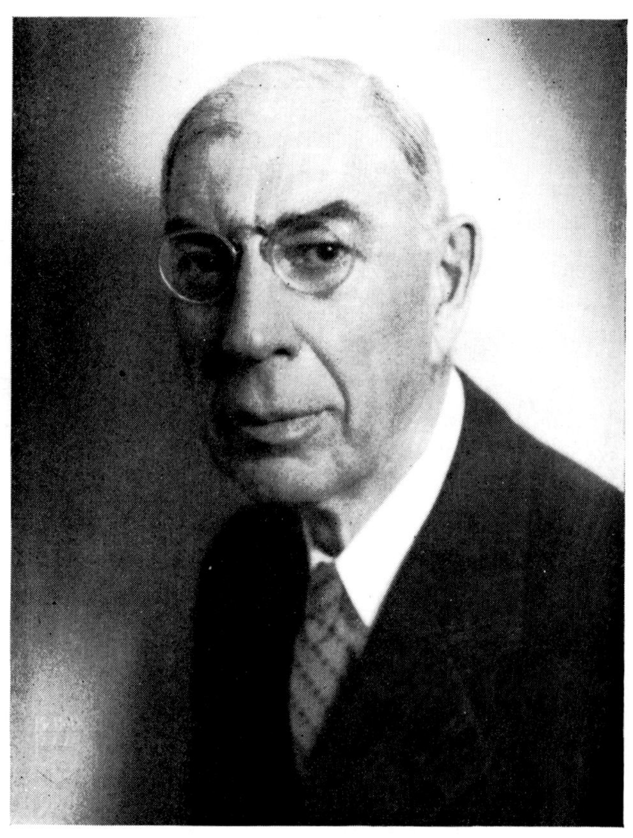

AUSTIN F. JAMES, D.D.S.
First President—1914 and 1915
American Academy of Periodontology

IV

Periodontia's Honor Roll

Now that the Ship of State (for such it seemed to its sponsors) has been launched with all sails set, let us pause long enough to take a look at that small group of men and women who, without chart or compass, succeeded in steering their frail bark into the uncertain Harbor of Success. Not only as voyagers on an unknown sea, but throughout the years which have elapsed since they set sail, these men and women have labored unceasingly for the ideal which possessed them and into which they breathed the breath of life on that May day in 1914. And lest we forget, let there be written on periodontia's Honor Roll, the names of those "who through long days of labor, and nights devoid of ease", pursued their course undaunted and unafraid:

GILLETTE HAYDEN: Founder with Dr. Spalding, of the American Academy of Periodontology. Member and Chairman of the Organization Committee. President 1916. Did outstanding work on the Dental Educational Bulletins. In coöperation with Dr. McCall, prepared the Record Charts. Leading spirit in the organization of the Academy. Executive ability of a high order. Fellow of the Academy.

In her untimely death, the Academy sustained one of its greatest losses. In recognition of Dr. Hayden's service to her profession and to the organization to which she gave so much of herself, the Journal of Periodontology has been dedicated to her memory—"for her pioneer efforts and selfless devotion in behalf of periodontia and the American Academy of Periodontology".

GRACE ROGERS SPALDING: With Dr. Hayden, founder of the American Academy of Periodontology. Member and Acting Secretary of the Organization Committee. Chairman of the Council 1915-16. Active as a member of the Council for approximately twenty years. Served as Secretary 1918-19 and President of the Academy 1923. Fellow of the Academy. Editor of the Journal of Periodontology since it was founded in 1929. Awarded Scroll of Honor at 25th anniversary meeting in 1938.

JOHN OPPIE MCCALL: One of the earliest members to support and encourage the Founders in the trying days that led up to the formation of the Organization Committee of which he later became a member. Drafted the first Constitution and By-laws. Member of the Nomenclature Committee where he rendered a service of distinct value. With Dr. Hayden, prepared the first Academy Record Charts. Fellow of the Academy. President 1917.

CLYDE M. GEARHART: An enthusiastic member of the Organization Committee. Took a firm stand against disbanding the newly formed organization in favor of a section in the National Dental Association. Also favored a limited membership. Arranged for the publication of the proceedings of the first annual meeting in the *Items of Interest*. Largely responsible for the program and entertainment at the meeting held in Washington, D. C., in November 1914. President 1922.

J. W. JUNGMAN: Member of Organization Committee. Acted as host to the Committee at its meeting February 21, 1914. Took a chief part in drafting the first Certificate of Fellowship.

A. C. HAMM: Member of Organization Committee. Took an active part by correspondence in the discussions which led up to the formation of the Organization Meeting. Was present at the meeting in Detroit in 1915.

J. HERBERT HOOD: Organization Committee member. Parliamentarian. Aided substantially in the final preparation of the Constitution and By-laws. President 1918. Secretary-Treasurer for several years in which office he rendered outstanding service.

Austin F. James: President first two years, 1914-15. Only president to serve for two terms. First to suggest the publication of a journal by the Academy in 1915. Coöperated in every activity for the advancement of periodontia. Rendered conspicuous service in the early days of the organization by the exercise of sound judgment at a time when it was most needed. Fellow of the Academy.

Andrew J. McDonagh: First Canadian member. Aided in bringing in other members from Canada, notably Drs. Box, Garvin, Webster, and Williams. Chairman of Scientific Investigation and Nomenclature Committees. Present nomenclature in periodontia largely the work of that Committee to which he and McCall made the fundamental contributions. Later made honorary member.

* * *

While others contributed to the advancement of the Academy and without whose coöperation and steady support, progress would have been less rapid, those whose names are here listed, deserve to be given first place when the Honor Roll of the Academy is made up. It was they who bore the burden and heat of the day "when as yet there was none of them". They were the pioneers who blazed the trail and made straight the pathway to success. In the face of many obstacles they held fast to their ideal—"held on through blame and faltered not at praise". To them the American Academy of Periodontology owes its existence.

V

Early Meetings

FIRST ANNUAL MEETING

The first annual meeting of the newly formed Academy of Oral Prophylaxis and Periodontology was held in Washington, D. C., November 5, 6, and 7, 1914, seventeen members being present. The meeting was called to order by the president, Dr. Austin F. James. Following a brief period of silent prayer, Dr. Gillette Hayden was appointed secretary in the absence of Dr. Charles P. Wood. The address of welcome was made by Dr. W. M. Simkins, President of the District of Columbia Dental Society, the response being made by President James. Report of several committees occupied the balance of the morning session. At the afternoon session the Vice-president, Dr. A. J. McDonagh took the chair and introduced Dr. James who read his Presidential Address, concluding with the statement: "You have made no mistake in selecting me as your first president if I am to be gauged by my enthusiasm. For I am with you in heart and in mind and in body and soul." General discussion of the

President's Address followed in which nine of those present participated, the statement being made that "75 per cent of the adult population have periodontal inflammation that finally results in the loss of some or all of the teeth, and 17 of us in all the United States are interested enough to be here today".

At the evening session Dr. Clarence J. Grieves addressed the meeting in "An Informal Talk on the Application of Oral Prophylaxis to a Large Hospital".

The morning of November 6 was given over to committee reports, chief among them being Dr. McDonagh's report on nomenclature and Dr. McCall's on scientific investigation. At the afternoon session the Academy members were the guests of Dr. Hrdlicka, Curator of the Division of Physical Anthropology, Smithsonian Institute. The evening of November 6 the Academy met at the George Washington University, Dental Department, where Dr. L. F. Kebler, Chief of the Drug Division, Bureau of Chemistry, Department of Agriculture, gave a lecture on "Dentifrices" in which he deprecated the use of such terms as "antiseptic and germicide" in the advertisements of dentifrices and the fact that there were those among the dental and medical professions who were willing to lend their names by indorsing such products.

A business meeting occupied the forenoon of November 7. In the afternoon the members were guests of Dr. and Mrs. Gearhart on a steamer trip to Mt. Vernon. The officers elected at the Organization Meeting on May 23 were continued in office.

SECOND ANNUAL MEETING

The second annual meeting of the Academy was held at the Hotel Statler, Detroit, September 20, 21, and 22, 1915, with twenty-one members in attendance as follows:

Andrew J. McDonagh	Austin F. James	R. R. Johnston
A. C. Hamm	J. W. Jungman	H. T. Stewart
Mary E. Alleyne	F. H. Skinner	A. E. Webster
John O. McCall	C. P. Wood	M. H. Garvin
Edna E. Noyes	J. J. Sarrazin	W. A. Price
C. M. Gearhart	N. S. Hoff	Grace Rogers Spalding
J. Herbert Hood	Paul R. Stillman	Gillette Hayden

The first session which convened on September 20 was opened with prayer, President James presiding. Minutes of previous meeting were read and approved. Treasurer's report showed balance on hand of $289.09. The President then read his address recommending among other things a program of education to include the profession and the public, and as soon as conditions would permit, the publication of a journal by the Academy. On motion the address was referred to a committee to be reported on at a later session.

The afternoon session was devoted to "General Business". The names of 15 candidates for membership were presented and having been previously approved by the Council, were elected. Dr. McCall proposed a consideration of what the field of the specialist in periodontia should consist. This provoked considerable discussion. Some expressed the opinion that it would be inexpedient to combine oral prophylaxis and "pyorrhea work" in a single specialty; that the former should be practiced as a preventive specialty for children and the latter as a specialty in "pyorrhea" to include all forms of restorative treatment. Others again expressed the belief that the specialty of periodontia should be limited largely to the treatment of periodontal diseases including the establishment of "normal articulation". No formal action was taken following the debate.

At the evening session Dr. Weston A. Price read a paper on A. "The Mechanism of Blood Stream Infections as Related to Mouth Lesions" and B, "Some Important Etiologic Factors in the Progressive Inflammatory Processes of the Gums". Illustrated by motion pictures.

All sessions on September 21 were held at the University of Michigan, Ann Arbor. The meeting was called to order by the President at 10 A.M. First order of business was the reading of the report on nomenclature by Dr. McDonagh. After considerable discussion it was voted that the Committee confer with a similar committee of the National Dental Association. The report of the Committee on the President's Address expressed approval of the recommendation for "free clinics one day each month, but so far as the publication of a monthly journal" was concerned "the committee was not ready to report". This was followed by considerable discussion pro and con in which the President joined by saying that "we have no warrant for existence unless we do more than just hold meetings. We have a mission to perform; first, to educate the profession, and second, the public". Following the business meeting the members were welcomed by Dr. N. S. Hoff, Dean of the Dental Department, University of Michigan. Inspection of the W. D. Miller collection and demonstrations in the Research Laboratory by Dr. Russell W. Bunting concluded the morning session.

At the afternoon session James G. Cumming, M.D., lectured on "The Bacteriology of the Mouth with Special Reference to Infection".

In Detroit, the forenoon of the following day, September 22, was given over to clinics, the clinicians being Dr. R. W. Bunting, Robert G. Owen, M.D., Frank Sladen, M.D., Dr. Edward B. Spalding, and several "informal clinics" by Academy members.

At the afternoon meeting officers for 1915 were elected as follows:

President, GILLETTE HAYDEN
First Vice-President, JOHN OPPIE MCCALL
Second Vice-President, J. J. SARRAZIN
Secretary, J. HERBERT HOOD
Treasurer, H. T. STEWART

To membership on the Council:

Gillette Hayden	Austin F. James
Grace Rogers Spalding	Andrew J. McDonagh
C. M. Gearhart	Paul R. Stillman
J. W. Jungman	

It was voted that election of officers should be held annually and that the president and vice-presidents should not be eligible for re-election. It was also voted that the president "submit his address to the Council for consideration one month before the annual meeting".

Following installation of officers the second annual meeting was adjourned to meet in 1916.

THIRD ANNUAL MEETING

At Pittsburgh, Pa., on July 20, 21, and 22, 1916, the American Academy of Oral Prophylaxis and Periodontology held its third annual meeting. No mention of the number in attendance is made in the Proceedings. That there was a substantial increase is probable since several new members had been elected at the Detroit meeting.

The proceedings were opened by a Council meeting at 9 o'clock on the morning of the first day, followed by President Hayden's address at 11 o'clock. This dealt largely with the necessity of providing proper charts for recording periodontal cases. The conditions to be recorded were listed as follows:

1. Condition of exposed and denuded root surfaces.
2. Condition of the periodontal tissues.
3. The occlusion.
4. Teeth missing.
5. Character of the operative work.
6. Personal care of the mouth.
7. Foci of infection.

The first item on the afternoon program was the report of the Committee on Scientific Investigation and Nomenclature in which the statement was made that "the terms adopted at this meeting will be presented to the profession in an effort to rid our literature of its present variety of unscientific terms". This was followed by a report of a Special Committee by Dr. Paul R. Stillman, as chairman, which contained "Resolutions to the President and members of the Research Institute of the National Dental Association"—one of the early, if not the earliest attempts by the Academy toward educating the body of general practitioners in the art and science of periodontology and more especially the members of the Research Institute. Though the Academy at this time was little more than two years old, it was already engaging in its task of education. Dr.

D. D. Smith had accepted an invitation to read a paper on Oral Prophylaxis at this session but was prevented from doing so by illness.

At a joint meeting with the American Society of Orthodontists at the evening session, Dr. Grace R. Spalding read a paper on "Practical Measures of Preventive Dentistry for the Orthodontist". This was followed by a paper by J. M. Rector, M.D. on "The Relation of Mouth Infections to Gastric and Intestinal Disorders".

A "Symposium on Periodontia as a Specialty", marked the opening of the morning session on July 21. Frank C. Pague of San Francisco, O. L. Hertig of Pittsburgh, and H. A. Pullen of Buffalo, were the essayists representing periodontia, general practice, and orthodontia respectively. Later in the session Dr. K. G. Knoche of Chicago read a paper on "Bridgework in Cases of Periodontoclasia".

The afternoon session was given over to social activities and the evening to a dinner for the members of the Academy, their wives, and guests—the first mention made of the annual dinners which have since become so popular a feature of Academy programs.

Clinics featured the morning session of July 22 in which ten participated. This was followed by a report of the Council and the election of officers, namely:

President, JOHN O. MCCALL
First Vice-President, M. H. GARVIN
Second Vice-President, R. R. JOHNSTON
Secretary-Treasurer, J. HERBERT HOOD

The Third Annual Meeting of the American Academy of Oral Prophylaxis and Periodontology, now fairly launched on its course, was adjourned to meet in New York in 1917 in connection with the National Dental Association. This marks the beginning of meetings in connection with the National Dental Association (which became the American Dental Association in 1922)—a custom which, with some exceptions, (to be noted later), has been followed since.

It has been thought best to give in some detail this history of the first three meetings of the Academy when it was still feeling its way through a maze of uncertainty, confusion and differing opinions. That out of it there should have emerged an organization such as the American Academy of Periodontology, is a matter of the utmost importance, for it focused attention on a group of diseases which had hitherto been regarded as more or less incurable. No longer ago than 1915 The Research Institute of the National Dental Association referred to "Pyorrhea Alveolaris" as an "almost incurable disease" for which "there is no positive cure . . .". It was to combat such statements that brought about the appointment of the Special Committee previously referred to.

VI

Later Meetings

From 1914 to 1941 the Academy has held annual meetings. With some exceptions (1921, 1924, 1926, 1930) these meetings have been held in connection with the American Dental Association, usually the last three days of the preceding week. This has been done to facilitate attendance at both meetings with a minimum of inconvenience to its members.

In 1926 the Academy met in New York in the week preceding the meeting of the International Dental Congress in Philadelphia. The responsibility for organizing the section on periodontia at the Congress had been delegated to the Academy and many of its members were in attendance. It was at these meetings in New York and Philadelphia that Dr. Bernard Gottlieb, then a resident of Vienna, took a prominent part in the proceedings and became known personally to many of the Academy members. Since then Dr. Gottlieb has become a citizen of the United States and one of the Academy's most distinguished members.

Beginning in 1942 and through 1945, annual meetings were discontinued because of war conditions except for an abbreviated meeting at Chicago in 1943. Council meetings, however, for the transaction of business have been held during each of these years. A list of these annual meetings with date, where held and name of president, is as follows:

1914—Washington, D. C.	Austin F. James
1915—Detroit, Mich.	Austin F. James
1916—Pittsburgh, Pa.	Gillette Hayden
1917—New York, N. Y.	John Oppie McCall
1918—Chicago, Ill.	J. Herbert Hood
1919—New Orleans, La.	Jules J. Sarrazin
1920—Boston, Mass.	Andrew J. McDonagh
1921—New York, N. Y.	Paul R. Stillman
1922—Cincinnati, Ohio	Clyde M. Gearhart
1923—Cleveland, Ohio	Grace Rogers Spalding
1924—Atlanta, Ga.	Olin Kirkland
1925—Louisville, Ky.	Arthur H. Merritt
1926—New York, N. Y.	M. Harry Garvin
1927—Detroit, Mich.	Carlos H. Schott
1928—Minneapolis, Minn.	Justin D. Towner
1929—Washington, D. C.	Julian Smith
1930—Colorado Springs, Colo.	Clyde C. Sherwood
1931—Memphis, Tenn.	Carl W. Hoffer
1932—Buffalo, N. Y.	Harold J. Leonard
1933—Chicago, Ill.	Benjamin Tishler
1934—St. Paul, Minn.	M. Monte Bettman
1935—New Orleans, La.	Walter H. Scherer
1936—San Francisco, Calif.	Haidee Weeks
1937—Atlantic City, N. J.	Edward B. Spalding

1938—St. Louis, Mo.	Clayton H. Gracey
1939—Milwaukee, Wis.	Alvin W. Bryan
1940—Cleveland, Ohio	Rudolph Kronfeld*
	Thomas B. Hartzell
1941—Houston, Texas	Isador Hirschfeld
1943—Chicago, Ill.	Robert L. Dement
1946—Birmingham, Ala.	Samuel R. Parks

Mention should be made also of the three Secretaries who each served for terms of seven or more years as Secretary-Treasurer and on the Local Arrangement Committees for the Annual Meetings, Dr. J. Herbert Hood, Dr. Clayton H. Gracey and Dr. Raymond E. Johnson. Much credit is due them for the continued development of this Academy.

There has been a steady growth in membership (which is by invitation only) throughout the years.

The first notice of Academy meetings appeared in the Journal of the National Dental Association in August, 1915, signed by Grace Rogers Spalding, Chairman of the Publicity Committee. This was the Detroit meeting. Notice of the Pittsburgh meeting is given in the Journal of the National Dental Association for May and August 1916, signed J. Herbert Hood, sec'y. (It is interesting to note that the Journal of the National Dental Association in 1916 was a quarterly consisting of 432 pages.) A more lengthy notice of the 1917 meeting with the list of officers and the names of some of those on the program, appeared in the National Dental Association Journal for October 1917—the month in which the New York meeting was held and the first in which the Academy met in connection with the National Dental Association.

From 1914 to 1918 inclusive, the Academy carried on under the title of the American Academy of Oral Prophylaxis and Periodontology. In 1919 this rather cumbersome title was dropped and its present name substituted.

Meanwhile the Academy's educational ferment was beginning to be felt within the profession, and in 1919 periodontia was wedded to orthodontia and made a section of the National Dental Association. This relationship was continued until 1929 when each became a section by itself. Prior to 1919, orthodontia had been grouped with prosthodontia, chemistry and allied subjects and welded into a section. (Periodontia had not at that time been recognized as a specialty.)

Since 1929, the section of periodontia of the American Dental Association has been the forum for discussion with the general practitioner of the many phases of periodontology. From the very beginning it has been one of the popular and best attended sections of the American Dental Association. Its educational value has been reflected in greater interest on the part of the family dentist in this aspect of dental practice and in the increasing number of those taking refresher courses in this field.

* Owing to the death of Dr. Kronfeld, the President-elect, Dr. Thomas B. Hartzell, presided.

No one can reflect upon the progress which has taken place in periodontia in the last quarter of a century in which the American Academy of Periodontology has been a prime mover, without a profound sense of satisfaction at what has been accomplished.

VII

Other Activities

1. EDUCATION

EDUCATION of the public in the care of the mouth and teeth in their relation to health in general has been one of the objectives of the Academy from its inception. This went hand in hand with education of the family dentist which was carried on by open meetings of the Academy, lectures, and discussions in the sections of the American Dental Association and as will be seen later, by the publication of the Journal of Periodontology.

Through a committee of which Drs. Gillette Hayden and Charles B. Fowlkes were hard working members, a series of articles—54 in number—were written in a popular style with catchy titles for publication in the public press. These were copyrighted by the Academy and found their way into thirty-three of the forty-eight states of this country and into nine foreign countries. The following titles will afford some idea of their scope and popular appeal: "Good Teeth to Last a Lifetime. Why we have Teeth. Hanging on to Life by the Teeth. Mastication for and With Good Teeth. Do Infected Teeth Ever Harm Eyes? Crooked Teeth are Worse than Bowlegs. Pyorrhea, What is it? Can Pyorrhea be Cured? How to Select Two Tooth Brushes", and others.

In addition to the above popularly written articles, a series of bulletins—8 in number—were prepared by the Academy. These were of a more ambitious nature, covered a wider range of information and were designed largely for adult use. Several of these were published by the American Dental Association where they could be purchased singly or in quantity for a few cents each. They were also reprinted and distributed by certain health agencies such as the Ohio Department of Health and the Federal Children's Bureau. One of the more ambitious of these and one having a wide distribution, was a bulletin entitled, "How to Build Sound Teeth", with a footnote stating it is "one of a series of bulletins on the teeth and their care for the information of the public". Since this was written in 1923 and its contents possibly forgotten, it might be worth while to note at this point the nature and scope of the information which it contained. It is stated by way of introduction that "It is the object of this bulletin to suggest what may be done to give Nature her chance to build sound teeth with sturdy supporting structures in the mouths of children." These are the headings to some of the 21 paragraphs of this bulletin:

Responsibility of Parents.
Essentials to Right Living.
General Diet Essentials for the Pregnant and Nursing Mother.
Tooth Decay During Pregnancy and Nursing Periods.
Care of Mother's Mouth.
Use of the Teeth.
Avoid Overeating.
The Child From Birth to Two Years.
The Child From Two to Six Years.
Ages Six to Eighteen.
The Temporary Teeth.
The First Permanent Molar.
Harmful Habits.
Mastication of Food.
Health Essentials.

The titles of other bulletins were:

"Children's Teeth—How to Use and Keep Them."
"What Bacteria do in the Mouth."
"The Masticating Machine."
"The Promotion of Health in the Mouth."
"Dietetics Applied to Oral Health."
"Home Care of the Mouth."
"The Treatment of Periodontoclasia."

Later the eight bulletins were combined in a booklet of which 500 copies were printed. Most of these were disposed of and found their way into lay publications in this country and abroad. It is doubtful if any educational matter of this nature was ever better done than that undertaken by these joint committees of the Academy.

In more recent years and as a part of the Academy's educational program, brief lecture courses in sciences related to periodontology have been given annually at the University of Michigan* to which all members of the Academy are invited. These courses have been well attended and have become a settled policy of the Academy.

2. JOURNAL OF PERIODONTOLOGY

Perhaps the most ambitious of the Academy's educational schemes and one that has been characterized as "one of its its finest accomplishments" is the publication of the Journal of Periodontology. The publication of such a journal had long been one of the objectives of the Academy, having been recommended by President James in his annual address in 1915. At the annual meeting at Washington in October 1929 the Committee on Dental Educational Bulletins of which Dr. Harold J. Leonard was then chairman, recommended the discontinuance of these bulletins and "the establishment of a periodically

* [The 1947 Seminar was given at the University of Minnesota—Ed.]

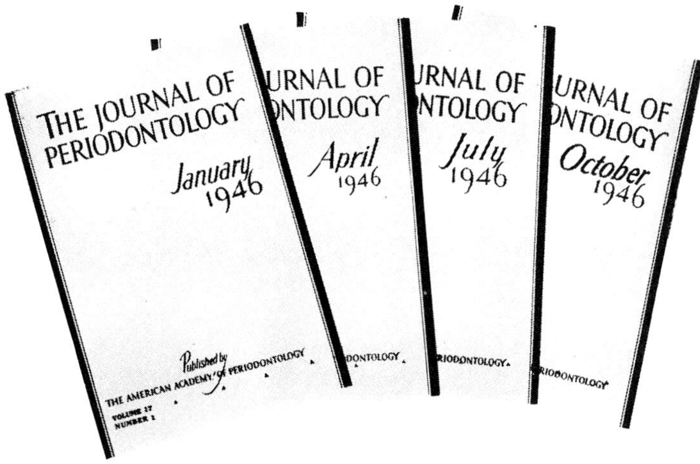

issued bulletin of information for the members of the Academy". At a luncheon conference of several of the members it was recommended that a "journal containing reviews of books and extracts of worth-while articles on periodontology and related sciences would best fill the need". It was also agreed that the Journal should be dedicated to the memory of Dr. Gillette Hayden whose death occurred on March 27, 1929. It was the desire of those present "to express in some permanent form their appreciation of her ideals" and "to stimulate and encourage the habit of reading and study of subjects relating to periodontology",—an idea which had been "uppermost in Dr. Hayden's mind for several years". Accordingly the following dedicatory inscription has appeared in most issues of the Journal since 1930:

> The Journal of Periodontology is lovingly dedicated to the memory of Doctor Gillette Hayden from whose achievements in the preparation of dental educational bulletins it is an outgrowth. Her selfless devotion and untiring efforts in behalf of the science of periodontology, the art of periodontia and the American Academy of Periodontology, have served as an inspiration to her close associates which can only be consummated by carrying onward the work for which she spent her life.

Having decided to publish a journal, the Council authorized the publication and financing of two issues in 1930. Dr. Grace Rogers Spalding was made editor, a position which she has held with distinction for seventeen years. The first issue is dated January 1930 and contains 26 pages with the caption, "Published twice annually—January and July by the American Academy of Periodontology".

"Owing to delay in receiving the abstracts" the second issue, (Vol. 2, No. 1) did not appear until January 1931, since which time up to 1945, when the Journal became a quarterly, it has been published twice each year.

In the Foreword to Vol. 2, No. 1 the statement is made that "This number marks the beginning of an attempt to bring together the scattered literature bearing on periodontology in a form available to students and practitioners. An effort has been made to list all books bearing on the subject, and to assemble all the current literature as abstracts, starting with Jan. 1927".

The bibliography—12 pages in length—covers the subject from 500 B.C. to 1930 A.D. Abstracts take up most of the remaining pages of this issue which have been a prominent feature in each of the 17 volumes.

While the subscription list is not large it has steadily grown and continues to increase each year. An encouraging feature is the number of foreign subscribers, a total of 76 in 26 countries including Australia, China, Denmark, Norway, Palestine, Portugal, Syria, and South Africa. This shows widespread interest in the science and art of periodontology and is most encouraging.

It has always been the policy of the Academy, acting through its Publication Committee to maintain the highest standards of professional journalism free from all taint of commercialism. It carries no advertisements. Academy proceedings along with other articles appear regularly in its pages, plus abstracts. In more recent years Dr. Harold J. Leonard has conducted a department under the title of "In Our Opinion", in which he invites certain members to express themselves on the question under discussion. This has proved interesting and instructive.

3. ACADEMY FELLOWSHIPS

Very early in its history the Academy took steps toward recognizing those who have "rendered conspicuous service of distinct and recognized value in the field of periodontology", (whether members of the Academy or not) by electing them Fellows of the Academy.

To this end a Fellowship Committee consisting of the president and six members has been set up. Nominations may be made by any member of the Academy which "shall be presented in writing to the Committee on Fellowships with evidence of the qualifications of the nominee". A three-fourths vote of the Academy is required for election.

The following are the names of those who have been elected to date:

Harold K. Box
Prof. W. J. Gies
Bernard Gottlieb
Gillette Hayden
Isador Hirschfeld
J. Herbert Hood
Austin F. James
Rudolf Kronfeld
John O. McCall
Arthur H. Merritt
John Dean Patterson
Grace Rogers Spalding
Paul R. Stillman
Justin D. Towner

4. THE AMERICAN BOARD OF PERIODONTOLOGY

Recognizing the need of adopting some means for raising the standard of practice in periodontia and for determining the qualifications of those engaged in its practice, the American Board of Periodontology was organized by the Academy in 1939 to meet these needs. The desirability of some such organization had long been a subject for consideration. Action had been delayed, however, because of the difficulty of defining periodontia and just what should and should not be included. No specialty in dentistry is more intimately related to general practice and none more dependent upon it for success. Thus such conditions as abnormalities in occlusion, defective contact points, loss of teeth and so forth, have to be considered in the practice of periodontia. And since some of those engaged in its practice included some or all of these in their treatment, who was to be recognized as periodontists? Such was the situation when in 1939 the Academy organized the American Board of Periodontology and incorporated it in the State of Illinois in 1940. Its object as set forth in the By-laws is, a. "To encourage the study, to elevate the standards, and to promote and improve the practice of periodontology. b. To determine the competence of those wishing to practice as periodontists, and to arrange, conduct and control investigations and examinations to determine the qualifications of such individuals as voluntarily apply for the certificate issued by the corporation. c. To grant and issue certificates in the field of periodontology to voluntary applicants, therefor, and to maintain a registry of holders of such certificates."

The members of the Board, six in number, are elected by the Academy for a term of three years each, so arranged that the terms of two expire each year. The officers consist of a Chairman, a Vice-Chairman, and a Secretary-Treasurer. Committees on Requirements, Examinations, Education, and Finance among others, are appointed by the Board. The duties of these committees are to "evaluate the credentials of all candidates . . . arrange facilities for examinations . . . investigate and offer recommendations as to the teaching facilities and curriculums of institutions engaged in dental instruction and clinical work in periodontology".

Candidates for certification must be members of the American Dental Association or its equivalent if foreigners; graduates from an acceptable dental school in the United States or Canada; of high ethical and professional standing; who have spent five or more years in the practice of dentistry largely devoted to periodontology; must present proof of postgraduate work in dentistry and submit a list of papers and books published by the candidate.

Prior to 1944, practitioners who for ten or more years had been recognized by their colleagues as proficient in the field of periodontology, or who for that length of time had been engaged in the teaching of periodontology and had contributed to its literature, might be considered by the Board as having satisfied the educational requirements and be entitled to certification. The fee for certification is $50 which includes the application fee of $25.*

Examinations are held annually, though provision is made for the holding of examinations more often when there are three or more candidates. These examinations are both clinical and written.

Those passing the examination are awarded a certificate which states that the candidate "having given satisfactory evidence of a high degree of knowledge, skill and experience in the science and art of periodontology is entitled by the authority of this Board to be enrolled as one who is Expert in the practice of Periodontia", signed by the six members of the Board.

Because of the difficulty of defining the boundaries of periodontia and to avoid possible misunderstanding, the word specialist was omitted from the

*[This has since been increased—Ed.]

certificate. Instead, the holder is certified as one who is *Expert in the practice of periodontia.*

It is the consensus of opinion of those who have taken an active part in organizing the American Board of Periodontology that the rules governing its actions can be more satisfactorily administered by those engaged in the practice of periodontia than by legislative enactment. Moreover, since those engaged in the practice of periodontia are to be found in every state in the Union, it would be difficult to obtain legislative action even if thought to be desirable.

Each year since its organization, candidates who have satisfied the Board of their qualification to practice periodontia have been added to the list of certified experts, though at present the number is not large. Again it may be said that the sole purpose of the Board has been to advance the standards and to promote and improve the practice of periodontia to the end that dentistry may be elevated and the public more satisfactorily served.

This brief history of the organization and activities of the American Board of Periodontology would not be complete without recording the debt which the Board owes to the efficient and unselfish leadership of Dr. Harold J. Leonard, who took an active part in its organization and in the formulation of its policy. He has acted as Secretary-Treasurer since its organization in 1939. Without his enthusiastic coöperation the Board could hardly have achieved its present success.

Conclusion

Periodontology represents one of the younger specialties in dentistry and can be said to have had its birth as a specialty in 1914 with the organization of the American Academy of Periodontology. This was something new. Throughout historic time there had been those who recognized certain diseases which affected the periodontal tissues, causing the teeth to loosen and fall out. There is abundant evidence that such diseases were prevalent among the Greeks, Phoenicians, Etruscans, Hebrews, Chinese, and Romans. Treatment of one kind or another was recommended for "strengthening the gums", usually of the most fantastic nature.

It was not until John M. Riggs (1810-1885) of Hartford, Conn., claimed that treatment was surgical rather than therapeutic that any progress can be said to have been made, in the treatment of these diseases. (By surgical treatment Riggs meant the use of instruments in contradistinction to therapeutic measures.) However, the first real step forward was taken with the formation of the American Academy of Periodontology in 1914. For the first time in history an organized attempt was made to bring order out of chaos in this field of dentistry. Committees on nomenclature, research, classification, education, etc., set to work to place periodontia on a scientific basis—something which up to this time had never been done.

In the foregoing pages are to be found the record of these achievements and the names of the principal actors. To them belongs the credit for having succeeded where others had failed. Theirs was the vision and theirs the reward that comes from a knowledge of work well done. "What further could be sought for or declared?"

Appendix B
Constitution and Bylaws of The American Academy of Periodontology

CONSTITUTION

ARTICLE I—NAME

The name of this organization shall be The American Academy of Periodontology, hereinafter called "the Academy" or "this Academy."

ARTICLE II—OBJECT

It shall be the object of this Academy to advance the art and science of periodontology, and by its application, maintain and improve the health of the public.

ARTICLE III—ORGANIZATION AND DISSOLUTION

This Academy is a nonprofit corporation organized under the laws of the State of Illinois.

If this corporation is dissolved at any time, no part of its funds or property may be distributed to, or among, its members. After payment of all indebtedness of this corporation the remaining funds or properties shall be used to foster the art and science of periodontology in a manner to be determined by the then-governing body of the corporation.

ARTICLE IV—MEMBERSHIP

The membership of this Academy shall consist of dentists and other persons whose qualifications and classifications shall be as established in Chapter I of the Bylaws.

ARTICLE V—DUES AND FEES

The dues and fees of the Academy shall be established in Chapter IX of the Bylaws.

ARTICLE VI—GOVERNMENT

SECTION 1. LEGISLATIVE BODY: The legislative body of this Academy shall be the General Assembly as provided in Chapter II of the Bylaws.

SECTION 2. EXECUTIVE BODY: The governing body of this Academy shall be the Executive Council as provided in Chapter IV of the Bylaws.

ARTICLE VII—OFFICERS

SECTION 1. ELECTIVE OFFICERS: The elective officers of this Academy shall be a President, a President Elect, a Vice President, an Immediate Past President, a Secretary and a Treasurer. All of these officers shall be elected under the provisions of Chapter II, Section 7 of the Bylaws.

SECTION 2. APPOINTIVE OFFICERS: The appointive officers of the Academy shall be an Executive Director, an Editor or Editors as shall be appointed by the Executive Council as provided in Chapter VIII of the Bylaws.

ARTICLE VIII—ANNUAL SESSION

The Annual Session of this Academy shall be composed of the annual session of the General Assembly as provided in Chapter II of the Bylaws and the annual scientific session as provided in Chapter XII of the Bylaws.

ARTICLE IX—AMERICAN BOARD OF PERIODONTOLOGY

This Academy shall sponsor the American Board of Periodontology as provided in Chapter X of the Bylaws.

ARTICLE X—JOURNAL

There shall be a journal of the American Academy of Periodontology as its official publication, as provided in Chapter XI of the Bylaws.

ARTICLE XI—ENDOWMENT FUNDS

This Academy may sponsor and receive endowment funds as memorials, for the support of its official publication, student loans and scholarships, and for other projects designed to promote the objective of the Academy.

ARTICLE XII—PRINCIPLES OF ETHICS

The Principles of Ethics and Code of Professional Conduct of this Academy shall be the *Principles of Ethics and Code of Professional Conduct* of the American Dental Association and shall govern the professional conduct of the members of this Academy.

ARTICLE XIII—AMENDMENTS

This Constitution may be amended at any annual session on recommendation of the Executive Council and three-fourths vote of the members of the General Assembly present and voting, provided that the proposed amendment has been submitted in writing to all voting members at least sixty (60) days prior to the date on which the vote is taken.

This Constitution also may be amended at any annual session on recommendation of the Executive Council and on unanimous vote of the members of the General Assembly present and voting, provided that the proposed amendment has been presented in writing at a previous meeting of said session.

BYLAWS

CHAPTER I—MEMBERSHIP

SECTION 1. CLASSIFICATION:

The members of this Academy shall be classified as follows:

(a) Active Members
(b) Associate Members
(c) Academic Members
(d) Student Members
(e) Nonresident Members
(f) Life Members
(g) Retired Members
(h) Honorary Members

SECTION 2. QUALIFICATIONS:

The qualifications for the various classifications of membership shall be as follows:

A. **Active Members.** Any dentist shall be eligible to be an Active Member who is licensed to practice in the United States, Puerto Rico or Canada and is a member in good standing of the American Dental Association, National Dental Association, Canadian Dental Association or a recognized Canadian provincial dental association and who meets at least one of the following qualifications:

1. is ethically qualified to announce as a specialist in periodontology according to the requirements of the American Dental Association and limits his practice to periodontology;
2. has continually been an Active Member of this Academy (or the American Society of Periodontists) since June 6, 1967; or
3. is engaged primarily in teaching and research in periodontology (or is a full time academic who has transferred from a teaching to an administrative position) with supplemental practice, if any, limited to periodontology.

A foreign-trained dentist residing in the United States, Canada or Puerto Rico who has completed advanced training in periodontics in a program accredited by the Commission on Dental Accreditation of the American Dental Association shall be eligible to be an Active Member even if he is not licensed to practice in one of those countries, provided that he meets the other criteria set forth above.

B. **Associate Members.** Any dentist shall be eligible to be an Associate Member who is a resident of the United States, Puerto Rico or Canada and is a member in good standing of the American Dental Association, the National Dental Association, the Canadian Dental Association or a recognized Canadian provincial dental association and is interested in the art and science of periodontology. However, no dentist who meets the qualifications to be an Active Member shall be eligible to be an Associate Member.

C. **Academic Members.** Any nondentist shall be eligible to be an Academic member who holds a doctoral degree or its equivalent and is engaged primarily in teaching or research in periodontology or in related areas and is not eligible for another category of membership in the Academy. There are no geographic restrictions on this category of membership.

D. **Student Members.** Any person shall be eligible to be a Student Member who is continuously enrolled in a training program in periodontology accredited by the Commission on Dental Accreditation of the American Dental Association. Student Members may remain such for up to two years after graduation, during which period their practices, if any, must be limited to periodontology. An extension of the two-year limitation may only be obtained by application to the Executive Council.

E. **Nonresident Members.** Any dentist residing outside of the United States, Puerto Rico or Canada shall be eligible to be a Nonresident Member who is a member of a recognized national dental association and interested in the art and science of periodontology.

F. Life Members. Any person shall be eligible for Life Membership who has been a member in good standing of a dues-paying classification of membership in the Academy for at least 25 years and has attained age 65.

G. Retired Members. A member in good standing of any dues-paying classification of membership in the Academy who completely retires from practice may be permitted to remain in the Academy as a Retired Member.

H. Honorary Members. Honorary Members shall be chosen from those persons who have made outstanding contributions to the art and science of periodontology.

No person who is in default with respect to any financial obligations to this Academy shall be eligible for admission to membership herein. Also, no person who is in violation of the *Principles of Ethics and Code of Professional Conduct* of the American Dental Association (or of analogous principles applicable to nonresidents of the United States) shall be entitled to admission to membership herein, except as specifically permitted by the Executive Council upon recommendation by the Committee on Membership. It is assumed that the Committee on Membership shall seek consultation from the Committee on Ethics when appropriate.

SECTION 3. PRIVILEGES OF MEMBERSHIP:

Members in good standing of the various classifications of membership shall be entitled to the following rights and privileges:

A. Active Members. Active Members shall be entitled to all rights and privileges of membership in the Academy including the right to vote, to make nominations, to hold office and to serve on all committees.

B. Associate, Academic, Student, Nonresident and Retired Members. Associate, Academic, Student, Nonresident and Retired Members shall be entitled to all the privileges of Active Members except the right to vote, to make nominations, to hold office or to serve on committees whose membership is limited to Active Members.

C. Life Members. Shall be entitled to the rights and privileges of membership attached to the classification of membership to which they belonged immediately prior to becoming Life Members.

D. Honorary Members. Shall be entitled to all the rights and privileges of an Active Member except the right to vote, to make nominations, to hold office or to serve on committees whose membership is reserved for Active members. Honorary Members shall in addition enjoy any greater rights and privileges attached to the classification of membership, if any, to which they belonged immediately prior to becoming Honorary Members.

SECTION 4. ADMISSION OF NEW MEMBERS:

A. Active, Associate, Academic and Nonresident Members. Any person wishing to become an Active, Associate, Academic or Nonresident Member shall complete a membership application and submit it to the Secretary of the Academy. The application must be accompanied by endorsements by two Active Members who shall attest to their personal knowledge of the applicant's good character, acceptable methods of practice or other relevant qualifications.

An applicant for Nonresident membership who is not in a position to obtain the endorsement of two Active Members may substitute endorsements as follows: (i)endorsement of the applicant's local or national dental association, or, if he is an academic, the endorsement of the head of his teaching institution may be substituted for one Active Member endorsement; and (ii)endorsement by an Associate, Academic or Nonresident Member may be substituted for the second Active Member endorsement.

An applicant for Associate Membership may substitute an endorsement from an Associate Member for one of the endorsements from Active Members.

All properly completed applications shall be referred by the Secretary to the Committee on Membership of the General Assembly. After consideration of the applicant's qualifications the Committee on Membership shall refer the application to the Executive Council, along with its recommendation for or against approval or for admission to a different membership classification than that applied for. If the Executive Council approves the application for admission to a different classification of membership, it shall nominate the applicant for election to that classification of membership by the General Assembly.

An election shall be held at the business session of the General Assembly for admission to membership. A list of all approved nominees shall be sent to all voting members of the Academy at least 30 days prior to the Annual Meeting. Nominees must receive the affirmative votes of at least three-fourths of all members present and voting in order to be admitted to membership.

All members-elect shall be sent a written invitation for membership in the Academy. The invitation must be accepted and any initiation fee paid within 30 days. Upon such acceptance and payment the member shall become entitled to all rights and privileges of membership.

B. **Student Members.** Any person wishing to become a Student Member shall submit an appropriate application to the Secretary, accompanied by an affidavit by his program director stating that he is a bona-fide full time student in a training program for the specialty of periodontics accredited by the Commission of Dental Accreditation of the American Dental Association.

All properly completed applications will be referred by the Secretary to the Executive Council. If the application is approved by the Executive Council the applicant's name shall be added to the official roster.

C. **Honorary Members.** The Executive Council may from time to time nominate candidates to become Honorary Members, whose names shall then be submitted to the General Assembly for approval.

SECTION 5. GOOD STANDING:

A member is considered to be in good standing so long as he has paid all dues and financial obligations to the Academy when due, is in compliance with the provisions of these By-laws concerning attendance requirements and certification of practice and his membership has not been suspended or terminated.

SECTION 6. ATTENDANCE REQUIREMENTS:

Active and Associate Members are required to attend at least one Annual Meeting during each three year period. There is no attendance requirement for the other classifications of membership.

In the event of illness or other extenuating circumstances a member may petition the Executive Council (by letter addressed to the Secretary) for an extension of the three year period, but such a petition must be submitted not later than 60 days after the last Annual Meeting at which his attendance would have been required in order to avoid noncompliance with the attendance requirements.

Reference shall be made to the provisions of this Section in all official notices of any Annual Meeting sent directly to members or published in the Academy's official publication.

SECTION 7. CERTIFICATION OF ELIGIBILITY:

All Active Members must certify by January 31st of each year the extent to which they practice periodontology. The payment of annual dues by a member of the Academy shall constitute a certification by such member that his practice, if any, is limited to periodontology if required by Section 2 above, and that such member otherwise continues to be eligible for membership in the classification in which he is enrolled.

It shall be the duty of each member of the Academy to advise the Secretary within 30 days of any change in his eligibility for his present classification of membership or mailing address.

SECTION 8. RECLASSIFICATION:

A. **Life Membership.** Members of the Academy meeting the applicable eligibility requirements may petition the Secretary for reclassification as a Life Member. After verifying the petitioner's eligibility, the Secretary shall notify the Executive Council that the petitioner has been reclassified.

B. **Retired Membership.** Members of the Academy meeting the applicable eligibility requirements may petition the Secretary for reclassification as Retired Members. Such petitions shall be referred by the Secretary to the Executive Council, which shall make a determination of the petitioner's eligibility.

C. **Other Classifications.** Members who become eligible for reclassification into other classifications of membership may complete an appropriate application for submission to the Secretary. Such applications will be treated as applications for new membership in the classification in question, except that supporting endorsements from Active Members will not be required if such endorsements were submitted in connection with a previous membership application. Once the reclassification is approved by the General Assembly, the member will become entitled to all of the privileges and responsibilities of the new membership classification upon payment of any differential in initiation fees between the new and the old membership classifications.

If a member loses his eligibility for his present classification of membership, the Committee on Membership may on its own initiative or at the request of the Secretary initiate a reclassification of the member into another membership classification for which he is eligible. The member shall be given notice of such proposed action and may voluntarily withdraw from membership in the Academy rather than accept the reclassification, or, if the member desires to contest the proposed action, request a hearing by the Membership Committee to be held during the Annual Meeting.

SECTION 9. WITHDRAWAL FROM MEMBERSHIP:

Membership may be voluntarily terminated by written request provided that the member requesting such termination is in good standing.

SECTION 10. SUSPENSION:

Members may be suspended from membership for a determined period of time in accordance with the disciplinary procedures provided for in Chapter XIII. During the period of suspension all membership privileges are revoked, except for eligibility for coverage under Academy insurance programs. All privileges are automatically restored at the conclusion of the suspension period.

SECTION 11. TERMINATION:

Membership will be automatically terminated upon notice to the member where: (a) a member has failed to pay his annual dues by May 1 (together with any applicable delinquency fine) or has defaulted on any other financial obligation due to the Academy and no petition for waiver of such dues or other obligation is pending in accordance with these bylaws: or (b) a member has failed to comply with the attendance requirements set forth in Section 6 above and no petition for an extension in accordance with such section is pending. Termination of membership means the complete loss of all privileges of membership. In those cases in which a timely petition for waiver or extension is pending in accordance with these bylaws, termination shall be postponed until the petition has been acted upon by the Executive Council.

A person may also be terminated from membership if he ceases to meet the qualifications for membership in the Academy. The Committee on Membership shall make an investigation concerning any change in a member's qualifications and shall make an appropriate recommendation to the Executive Council if it finds that reclassification or termination is in order. The Executive Council shall make a final decision with regard to terminations. Recommendations for reclassification shall be dealt with in accordance with the procedure provided for in Chapter I, Section 8.

Membership may also be terminated as a result of a disciplinary proceeding conducted in accordance with the provisions of Chapter XIII.

SECTION 12. REINSTATEMENT:

A person who voluntarily withdraws or whose membership has been terminated for failing to meet the attendance requirements set forth in Section 6 above shall be eligible for reinstatement without the payment of a new initiation fee if he submits an appropriate petition to the Secretary within two years from the date of withdrawal or termination, provided that he remains eligible for mem-

bership and that, in the latter case, he has attended at least one Annual Meeting in the interim (at which he has paid the nonmember registration fee). The Secretary (after verifying such attendance, if appropriate) shall refer all such petitions to the Committee on Membership, which shall submit the petition, together with its recommendation for or against reinstatement, to the Executive Council for a final decision.

Except as provided for in the preceding paragraph, any person who voluntarily withdraws or whose membership is terminated in accordance with Section 11 above who wishes to be readmitted to membership in the Academy will be subject to the same application procedure and requirements as for new members (including the payment of any applicable initiation fee).

SECTION 13. ELECTION TO FELLOWSHIP:

A member may be elected by the Executive Council to become a Fellow of the Academy in recognition of distinguished service. Election as a Fellow does not alter the person's membership status.

CHAPTER II—GENERAL ASSEMBLY

SECTION 1. NAME AND COMPOSITION:

The legislative body of this Academy shall be the General Assembly, which shall be composed of all voting members of the Academy.

SECTION 2. POWERS AND DUTIES:

The General Assembly shall have the following powers and duties:

(a) It shall be the supreme policy-making body of this Academy;

(b) It shall have the power to enact, amend and repeal the Constitution and Bylaws of this Academy, upon the recommendation of the Executive Council;

(c) It shall elect all new members of the Academy except Student Members and shall approve all reclassifications of members into classifications other than Life and Retired memberships;

(d) It shall approve all memorials made in the name of the Academy;

(e) It shall elect all Elected Officers except as otherwise provided by these Bylaws;

(f) It shall elect the members of all committees and boards of the Academy, except as otherwise provided in these Bylaws;

(g) It shall serve as the final appellate body from decisions of the Executive Council on any disciplinary action taken against a member of the Academy pursuant to Chapter XIII;

(h) It shall approve the annual budget of the Academy.

SECTION 3. MEETINGS:

A. **Annual Meeting.** The Annual Meeting of the General Assembly shall be held at the time and place determined by the Executive Council during the Annual Meeting of the Academy. Written notice thereof shall be given to all members of the academy who are eligible to attend not less than 10 nor more than 60 days before the dates thereof. Once such notice has been sent to the members, the meeting may only be postponed in the case of extreme emergency, as determined by a three-fourths vote of the Executive Council. Written notice of any such postponement shall be sent to all members.

B. **Special Meetings.** A Special Meeting of the General Assembly may be called by a two-thirds vote of the Executive Council at such time and place as the Council may determine. Written notice thereof shall be given to all members who are eligible to attend not less than 10 nor more than 60 days prior to the date thereof.

SECTION 4. QUORIUM:

Fifty voting members of the Academy shall constitute a quorum for the transaction of business at any meeting of the General Assembly.

SECTION 5. ORDER OF BUSINESS:

The Order of Business at the Annual Meeting of the General Assembly shall be determined in advance by the President of the Academy, subject to modification during the meeting by a majority vote of the members present and voting.

SECTION 6. RULES OF ORDER:

The rules contained in the latest revised edition of *Sturgis Standard Code of Parliamentary Procedure* shall govern the deliberations of the General Assembly, except where they conflict with the Constitution, Bylaws, or standing rules of the Academy.

SECTION 7. ELECTION PROCEDURES:

Whenever these Bylaws provide for the election of an officer or committee member of the Academy or Director of the American Board of Periodontology by means of mail ballots to be sent to the voting members of the Academy or of a District of the Academy, the following procedure shall be followed: By no later than March 1st the Executive Director shall send to each such voting member a list of the names of the candidates nominated by the nominating body provided for in the relevant section of these Bylaws, together with a notice explaining the procedure for nominating additional candidates by petition. Such candidates may be nominated by written petitions signed by at least ten voting members which are received by the Secretary of the Academy no later than May 1st. No nominee's name shall be included on an election ballot unless he has indicated in writing his willingness to serve if elected.

By no later than June 1st the Executive Director shall send a mail ballot setting forth the names of all candidates to each voting member of the General Assembly or of the District concerned. The ballot shall conform to the design principles incorporated in absentee ballots used in the election of the President of the United States, and shall be accompanied by biographical sketches of each candidate. Ballots shall be returned to the indicated address by no later than August 1st. The Executive Council shall appoint tellers for the counting of ballots. The candidate for a particular office or position receiving the greatest number of votes shall be declared elected. In the event of a tie, the Executive Council shall cast the deciding ballot. The announcement of the results of the election and the installation of the successful candidates in office shall take place at the next annual meeting of the Academy.

The returned ballots and a list of the ballots issued shall be maintained in confidence and shall be destroyed 30 days after the ballot return date. A majority vote of the Executive Council shall be required for the examination of such materials. The General Assembly shall have final authority concerning any question of election procedure or irregularity. All reasonable expenses incurred in holding the elections shall be paid out of Academy funds.

SECTION 8. REFERENDUM:

The General Assembly may by a majority vote of those members present and voting at any meeting determine that a question relating to the administration or policies of the Academy should be submitted to the voting members of the Academy in the form of a referendum. Appropriate ballots, including detailed information relative to the proposal, shall then be mailed to all voting members by the Secretary. Ballots must be received in the Central Office within 60 days from that date on which the ballots are distributed in order to be counted. A majority vote of no less than thirty percent of the total ballots mailed shall be required for adoption of the proposal.

CHAPTER III—COMMITTEES OF GENERAL ASSEMBLY

SECTION I. TYPES OF COMMITTEES:

The committees of the General Assembly shall consist of standing committees, special committees and the Committee on Credentials.

SECTION 2. STANDING COMMITTEES:

The General Assembly shall have six standing committees designated as follows:

(a) Committee on Constitution and Bylaws.

(b) Committee on Membership.
(c) Committee on Education.
(d) Committee on Research in Periodontology.
(e) Committee on Ethics.
(f) Committee on Nominations.

SECTION 3. COMPOSITION:

A. Committee on Nominations. The Committee on Nominations shall be composed of nine members consisting of (a) the Chairman of the Executive Council, (b) four additional members of the Executive Council appointed by the Chairman of the Executive Council for staggered two-year terms (no two of which additional members shall be from the same district), and (c) four other Active Members elected as set forth below. The Chairman of the Executive Council shall serve as chairman of the committee, but shall vote only in the event of a tie. The chairman shall appoint a vice chairman for a one-year term from among the other members of the Committee, who shall preside in the chairman's absence.

The four Active members referred to in clause (c) above shall be elected for one year terms as follows: in even numbered years each of the four even-numbered districts shall elect one representative, and in odd-numbered years each of the four odd-numbered districts shall elect one representative. At least two candidates for each such position shall be nominated by the District Nominating Committees of the Districts involved during the Annual Meeting of the Academy preceding the election.

B. Other Standing Committees. All other standing committees, with the exception of the Committee on Membership, shall be composed of five Active Members elected by the General Assembly by mail ballot for staggered three-year terms. Members may serve for two full consecutive three-year terms. In addition, the President of the Academy shall be an *ex officio* member of all such committees. In the case of new committees, two of the initial members shall be elected for one-year terms, two for two-year terms, and one for a three-year term.

The Committee on Membership shall be composed of eight Active Members, one from each district, nominated and elected by their respective districts for staggered three year terms. At least two candidates for each such position shall be nominated by the District Nominating Committee of the Districts involved during the Annual Meeting of the Academy preceding the election.

By no later than February 1st of each year the Committee on Nominations and the District Nominating Committees shall meet and submit to the Executive Director a list of candidates for vacancies on their respective committees. The procedures for nomination of additional candidates by petition and election by mail ballot set forth in Chapter II, Section 7 shall then apply.

The chairman of each such committee shall be appointed from among the members of the committee for a one year term by the President of the Academy with the consent of the Executive Council.

SECTION 4. POWERS AND DUTIES:

A. General. All Committees shall be governed by the provisions of these Bylaws. It shall be the duty of all Committees as an integral part of the Academy to work in cooperation with and report to the Executive Council and to be under its supervision for the accomplishment of the aims and purposes of the Academy. No resolution of any committee shall be deemed to establish the policy of the Academy until it has been approved by the Executive Council and/or the General Assembly.

B. Committee on Constitution and Bylaws. The Committee on Constitution and Bylaws shall formulate and submit to the Executive Council wording for all proposed amendments to the Constitution and Bylaws. It shall be within the purview of the committee to examine the Constitution and Bylaws and recommend changes in the wording thereof to the Executive Council in order to resolve conflicts between provisions, clarify ambiguities or make other technical improvements therein.

C. Committee on Membership: The Committee on Membership shall develop programs for the promotion of membership in the Academy and shall recommend applicants for membership.

D. Committee on Education. The Committee on Education shall confer with the administrators and program directors of dental schools, institutions having advanced training programs in periodontics and the Council on Dental Education to promote predoctoral and advanced teaching on periodontology. It shall conduct a continuing study of education in periodontology, make reports on same to the Executive Council and develop special activities in this field for the members of the Academy.

E. Committee on Research in Periodontology. The Committee on Research in Periodontology shall conduct a continuing study of research in periodontology, make annual recommendations on same to the Executive Council for review and develop the Academy's participation in the field.

F. Committee on Ethics. The Committee on Ethics shall provide advisory opinions regarding the interpretation of the *Principles of Ethics and Code of Professional Conduct* of the American Dental Association and shall conduct preliminary investigations and make reports to the Executive Council concerning disciplinary actions against members of the Academy in accordance with the provisions of Chapter XIII.

G. Committee on Nominations. The Committee on Nominations shall nominate candidates for offices and positions which are to be filled by election by the voting members unless otherwise specified by these Bylaws.

SECTION 5. SPECIAL COMMITTEES:

The General Assembly may create special committees for specified terms of not more than one year. The number and category of members, the manner of their appointment and the functions of such committees shall be as set forth in the resolutions creating them. The President shall serve as an *ex officio* member of all such committees.

SECTION 6. COMMITTEE ON CREDENTIALS:

At least 20 days in advance of the Annual Meeting the President shall appoint three Active Members to serve as Committee on Credentials at the meeting. The Committee on Credentials shall pass on questions arising at meetings of the General Assembly concerning voting eligibility.

SECTION 7. ACTIONS BY COMMITTEES:

A. Action at Meetings. Meetings of committees may be called by the Chairman by giving all members at least 10 days notice of the time, place and purpose thereof. A majority of the members of the committee shall constitute a quorum. A majority vote of members present at a meeting at which a quorum exists shall be required for adoption of resolutions and reports of the committee.

B. Action Without a Meeting. A Committee may also adopt reports and resolutions without a meeting if after circulation of a written proposal to all members of the committee a majority of such members approve the proposal in writing.

SECTION 8. VACANCIES:

The President of the Academy shall appoint a member to fill any vacancy which occurs in a committee of the General Assembly, until a successor can be elected or appointed in accordance with the applicable Bylaw procedure.

CHAPTER IV—EXECUTIVE COUNCIL

SECTION 1. NAME AND COMPOSITION:

The supreme executive body of this Academy shall be the Executive Council (sometimes referred to herein as the "Council") which shall be composed of the President, President Elect, Vice President, Secretary, Treasurer, and the Immediate Past President of the Academy, all *ex officio*, plus twenty-one District Executive Council Members who shall be elected in accordance with the procedures set forth in Chapter VI below and one non-voting Associate Member representative appointed to a three year term by the President subject to approval by the Executive Council. The Associate Member representative may not serve for more than two consecutive full terms.

All Past Presidents of the Academy shall have the right to participate in the meetings of the Executive Council but, except for the Immediate Past President, shall not have the right to vote.

SECTION 2. POWERS AND DUTIES:

The Executive Council shall manage the property and affairs of the Academy, subject to the provisions of the Constitution, these Bylaws and any pertinent resolutions of the General Assembly. Between meetings of the General Assembly the Executive Council shall have the power to establish and interim policies for the Academy, which policies shall be reported to the General Assembly for ratification at the next meeting thereof.

SECTION 3. TERMS OF OFFICE:

Council Members who serve on the Council by virtue of being officers of the Academy shall continue to serve so long as they hold their positions as officers. The terms of the District Executive Council Members shall be as set forth in Chapter VI.

SECTION 4. OFFICERS OF EXECUTIVE COUNCIL:

The President of this Academy shall serve as Chairman of the Executive Council and the Secretary of this Academy as Secretary of the Executive Council.

SECTION 5. VACANCIES:

Vacancies in District Council Seats shall be filled as set forth in Chapter VI. Vacancies in the seats held *ex officio* by the Elected Officers of the Academy shall be filled by their successors in office, where such are provided for by the provisions of Chapter VII, Section 5.

SECTION 6. MEETINGS:

A. **Annual Meeting.** The Executive Council shall meet annually immediately prior to the annual meeting of the General Assembly.

B. **Special Meetings.** A special meeting of the Executive Council may be called by the Chairman with the concurrence of two additional Council members and must be called by the Chairman upon the written request of six or more members. Members shall be given at least 10 days notice of any special meeting.

SECTION 7. QUORUM:

Two-thirds of the Executive Council in office shall constitute a quorum for the transaction of business.

SECTION 8. RULES OF ORDER:

The rules contained in the latest revised edition of *Sturgis Standard Code of Parliamentary Procedure* shall govern the deliberations of the Executive Council, except where inconsistent with the Constitution or Bylaws of the Academy.

SECTION 9. ACTION WITHOUT A MEETING:

The Executive Council may conduct its affairs by telephone or by mail when the President, or in his absence the President Elect, determines that the best interest of the Academy requires such action. All actions taken shall be presented for ratification at the next session of the Executive Council.

CHAPTER V—COMMITTEES OF THE EXECUTIVE COUNCIL

SECTION 1. TYPES OF COMMITTEES:

The committees of the Executive Council shall consist of standing committees and special committees.

SECTION 2. STANDING COMMITTEES:

The Executive Council shall have five standing committees as follows:

(a) Ad Interim Committee.
(b) Committee on Budget and Audit.
(c) Committee on Personal Membership Matters.
(d) Committee on the Annual Meeting.
(e) Committee on Professional Relations.

SECTION 3. COMPOSITION:

A. Ad Interim Committee. The Ad Interim Committee shall consist of the President, the President-Elect, the Vice President, the Immediate Past President, Secretary, Treasurer and two additional members of the Executive Council to be appointed annually by the chairman of the Council. The President shall serve as chairman of the Ad Interim Committee and the Secretary of the Academy shall serve as secretary of the committee.

B. Committee on Budget and Audit. The Committee on Budget and Audit shall consist of the President Elect, the Secretary and Treasurer of the Academy and two additional members of the Executive Council appointed annually by the Council.

The Chairman of the Budget and Audit Committee shall be appointed annually by the President of the Academy with the consent of the Executive Council from among the members of the Committee.

C. Committee on Personal Membership Matters. The Committee on Personal Membership Matters shall consist of the Secretary of the Academy plus two additional members of the Executive Council appointed annually by the Council. The Secretary shall serve as chairman of the committee.

D. Committee on the Annual Meeting. The Committee on the Annual Meeting shall consist of three Active Members, one of which shall be appointed annually by the Vice President for a three-year term. The senior member of the committee shall serve as chairman.

E. Committee on Professional Relations. The Committee on Professional Relations shall consist of eight Active Members appointed by the Executive Council for staggered three-year terms. Members may serve for two full consecutive three-year terms.

SECTION 4. POWERS AND DUTIES:

A. General. All committees shall be governed by the provisions of these Bylaws. It shall be the duty of all committees as an integral part of the Academy to work in cooperation with and report to the Executive Council as a whole and to be under its supervision for the accomplishment of the aims and purposes of the Academy. No action, report or recommendation of any committee shall be effective unless adopted by the Executive Council.

B. Ad Interim Committee. The Ad Interim Committee shall exercise the power and authority of the Executive Council between meetings of the Council when the chairman of the committee deems that such action is essential to the management of the Academy. All actions taken by the committee shall be presented for ratification at the next session of the Executive Council.

C. Committee on Budget and Audit. The Committee on Budget and Audit shall prepare an annual budget showing the revenues and expenditures of the Academy and it shall audit, or cause to be audited, the financial records of the Academy on an annual basis. The committee shall make an annual report to the Executive Council on its activities.

D. Committee on Personal Membership Matters. The Committee on Personal Membership Matters shall consider members' petitions for waivers of dues or extensions of attendance requirements which are referred to it by the Secretary and shall recommend appropriate action to the Executive Council. The committee shall also consider such additional matters as the Council may refer to it from time to time.

E. Committee on the Annual Meeting. The Committee on the Annual Meeting shall be in charge of all arrangements for the Annual Meeting of the Academy, including the annual scientific session (see Chapter XII).

F. Committee on Professional Relations. The Committee on Professional Relations shall prepare programs and materials for developing increased interest and better understanding by the dental profession in the area of periodontology.

SECTION 5. SPECIAL COMMITTEES:

Special committees of the Executive Council may be created by the Council as it deems appropriate. Members of such committees shall be appointed by the Council from among the members of the Academy for terms not exceeding one year. The number of committeemen and the functions of such committees shall be as set forth in the Council resolutions creating them. The President shall be an *ex officio* member of all such committees. Each special committee shall make an annual report on its activities and recommendations to the Executive Council and such interim reports as the Council may request.

SECTION 6. ACTIONS BY COMMITTEES:

A. Action at Meetings: Meetings of committees may be called by the chairman by giving all members at least 10 days notice of the time, place and purpose thereof. A majority of the members present at a meeting at which a quorum exists shall be required for adoption of resolutions and reports of the committee.

B. Action Without a Meeting. A committee may also adopt reports and resolutions without a meeting if after circulation of a written proposal to all members of the committee the proposal is approved by a majority of such members in writing.

SECTION 7. VACANCIES:

Vacancies in committee positions held *ex officio* by officers of the Academy shall be filled by their successors in office. In the event of any other vacancy in a committee of the Executive Council the Chairman of the Council shall appoint an interim successor to serve until the next meeting of the Council, when a successor shall be appointed for the unexpired term.

CHAPTER VI—DISTRICT ORGANIZATION

SECTION 1. PURPOSE:

The United States, Puerto Rico and Canada shall be divided into eight districts for the purpose of providing direct regional and sectoral representation of the voting members of the Academy in the election of the District Members of the Executive Council and the members of the Nominating Committee for the American Board of Periodontology.

SECTION 2. DEFINITION OF DISTRICTS:

The membership of the Academy shall be divided into eight Districts, as follows:

District 1. Members residing in Connecticut, Maine, Massachusetts, New Hampshire, Rhode Island, Vermont, Province of Quebec and the Maritime Provinces of Canada.

District 2. Members residing in Delaware, District of Columbia, Maryland, Pennsylvania, West Virginia, and the following cities and counties of the State of Virginia: Alexandria, Falls Church, Fairfax City, Vienna, Arlington County, Fairfax County, Prince William County, and Loudon County.

District 3. Members residing in Alabama, Florida, Georgia, Kentucky, Mississippi, North Carolina, South Carolina, Tennessee and Virginia with the exception of the following cities and counties: Alexandria, Falls Church, Fairfax City, Vienna, Arlington County, Fairfax County, Prince William County and Loudon County.

District 4. Members residing in Illinois, Indiana, Iowa, Kansas, Michigan, Minnesota, Missouri, North Dakota, Ohio, South Dakota, Wisconsin, Province of Ontario and Province of Manitoba.

District 5. Members residing in Arkansas, Colorado, Louisiana, Nebraska, Oklahoma, Puerto Rico and Texas.

District 6. Members residing in Alaska, Arizona, California, Hawaii, Idaho, Montana, Nevada, New Mexico, Oregon, Utah, Washington, Wyoming, Province of British Columbia, Province of Alberta and Province of Saskatchewan.

District 7. Members residing in New Jersey and New York.

District 8. Federal Dental Services. Members in the employment of the Federal Government including all branches of federal service, both civillian and military.

SECTION 3. ANNUAL CAUCUS.

A. General Each district shall hold caucus during the period of the Annual Meeting of the Academy. Notice of the time, place and purpose of the caucus shall be mailed to each voting member in the District at least 30 days before the caucus. The senior District Council member from the District shall preside over the caucus. The Executive Council may establish rules consistent with these Bylaws for the conduct of the caucus. The Council shall also cause an agenda for each caucus to be made available to the members prior to the caucus, which agenda may be modified by a majority vote of the members present at the caucus.

B. Election of the District Nominating Committee. During its annual caucus each District shall elect a District Nominating Committee for the purpose of nominating candidates for the seats on the Executive Council, the Membership Committee, the Nominating Committee and the Nominating Committee for the Board that are assigned to the District. The District Nominating Committee shall consist of a chairman and four committeemen, all of whom shall serve for one-year terms. All such committeemen shall be members of the District concerned.

C. Other Actions. The District caucuses may informally consider other matters relating to the purposes and aims of the Academy, but no resolution of any causes with respect to any such matter shall be binding upon Academy.

SECTION 4. QUALIFICATIONS AND TERMS OF DISTRICT EXECUTIVE COUNCIL MEMBERS:

Each District Executive Council Member must be an Active Member of the Academy in good standing and must be a member of the District which he represents. District Executive Council Members shall be elected for terms of three years. No member may serve for more than two consecutive full terms. The terms of Executive Council Members from Districts represented by more than one member shall be staggered in accordance with a schedule which the Executive Council shall adopt.

SECTION 5. ADDITIONAL DUTIES OF DISTRICT EXECUTIVE COUNCIL MEMBERS:

In addition to the duties imposed on all members of the Executive Council by the provisions of Chapter IV above, each District Executive Council Member shall serve as liaison between the governing bodies of the Academy and the members of his District. As such he shall be responsible for the dissemination of information from the Academy to the District members under the direction and supervision of the Executive Council.

SECTION 6. APPORTIONMENT OF EXECUTIVE COUNCIL SEATS AMONG DISTRICTS:

The twenty-one (21) District seats of the Executive Council shall be apportioned among the eight Districts using the "Method of Least Proportional Error" on the basis of each District's proportionate representation of the voting members of the Academy. Every three years the Executive Council shall review the distribution of voting members among Districts and shall reapportion the District Council seats among the Districts if required in order to maintain equal representation of voting members. The Executive Council shall have the power to provide for interim one- or two-year terms for newly elected District Executive Council Members in order to maintain an even staggering of District Council Member terms in Districts with an increased number of seats. In Districts suffering a decrease in the number of such seats, the Executive Council may provide for the premature expiration of the terms of District Executive Council Members currently in office, if necessary. In eliminating such seats the Council shall be guided by the principle of allowing the District Executive Council Members with the most seniority to complete their full terms, within the context of maintaining an even staggering of the terms of the members in the District on an overall basis.

SECTION 7. NOMINATION OF CANDIDATES FOR DISTRICT EXECUTIVE COUNCIL SEATS:

During the Annual Meeting of the Academy preceding any election to fill a vacancy in a District Council seat, the District Nominating Committee of the District concerned shall meet to nominate two or more candidates for each such seat. The Committee shall give due consideration to the need for full and fair geographic representation of all members in the District. A written report containing the names of the nominees shall be submitted to the Executive Director by December 1st. If such a list of nominees is not received by such date, the senior District Executive Council Member for the District concerned shall call a meeting of the District Nominating Committee which shall nominate candidates and submit a list thereof to the Executive Director not later than January 1st. Any expenses associated with such a meeting shall be borne by the District concerned rather than by the Academy. Additional candidates may be nominated by petition of ten voting members of the District concerned in accordance with the procedure described in Chapter II, Section 7.

An election shall be held by an appropriate mail ballot for each District concerned in accordance with the procedures set forth in Chapter II, Section 7.

SECTION 8. VACANCIES IN DISTRICT EXECUTIVE COUNCIL SEATS:

In the event of a vacancy in any District Council seat the President of the Academy shall appoint an Active Member from the District in question to serve until a successor can be elected by the District to fill the unexpired term.

SECTION 9. RECALL OF DISTRICT EXECUTIVE COUNCIL MEMBER:

Any District Executive Council Member may be recalled as provided in the Procedures for Recall of District Executive Council Members and Elected Officers incorporated herein by reference.

SECTION 10. NOMINATION AND ELECTION OF COMMITTEE MEMBERS BY THE DISTRICTS:

During the Annual Meeting of the Academy, the District Nominating Committee of the district concerned shall meet. They shall propose two or more candidates for any vacancy on the Membership Committee, the Nominating Committee, and on the Nominating Committee for the Board. A written report containing the names of the nominees shall be submitted to the Executive Director by December 1st. If such a list of nominees is not received by such date, the senior District Executive Council Member for the District concerned shall call a meeting of the District Nominating Committee, which shall nominate candidates and submit a list thereof to the Executive Director not late than January 1st. Any expenses associated with such a meeting shall be borne by the District concerned rather than by the Academy. Additional candidates may be nominated by petition of ten voting members of the District concerned in accordance with the procedure described in Chapter II, Section 7.

CHAPTER VII - ELECTED OFFICERS

SECTION 1. DESIGNATIONS:

The Elected Officers of the Academy shall be a President, a President Elect, a Vice President, an Immediate Past President, a Secretary, and a Treasurer.

SECTION 2. DUTIES:

A. **President.** The President shall preside over all meetings of the General Assembly, at which he shall cast the deciding ballot in the case of a tie vote, appoint judges and tellers for all elections and perform such other duties as custom and parliamentary usage prescribe. He shall present an annual written report to the Academy on the state of the Academy. He shall serve as the chairman of the Executive Council.

   He shall perform such other duties as are set forth elsewhere in these Bylaws.

B. **President Elect.** The President Elect shall assume that duties of the President in his absence and shall by actively aiding the President acquaint himself as thoroughly as possible with the duties of that office in preparation for his succession thereto.

C. **Vice President** The Vice President shall assume the duties of President in the absence of both the President and President Elect. He shall also assist the President and President Elect in the performance of their duties and shall be consulted on committee appointments to be made by the President.

D. **Immediate Past President.** The Immediate Past President shall advise the President in the performance of the duties of that office.

E. **Secretary.** The Secretary shall serve as secretary of the General Assembly and the Executive Council and shall prepare all official minutes and reports of proceedings. He shall be the custodian of all records of the Academy except those pertaining to the office of the Treasurer and shall maintain a list of members of the Academy by District. He shall make an annual report of his activities to the General Assembly and to the Executive Council and shall perform such other duties as are prescribed by these Bylaws or by resolution of the Executive Council or General Assembly.

F. **Treasurer.** The treasurer shall be responsible for the custody of all monies, securities and other financial assets of the Academy and shall hold, invest or disburse same subject to the direction of the Executive Council. He shall perform such other duties as are prescribed by these Bylaws or by resolution of the Executive Council or General Assembly.

SECTION 3. QUALIFICATIONS AND TERM OR OFFICE:

Only Active Members of the Academy may serve as Elected Officers. All Elected Officers shall assume office at the close of the Annual Meeting of the Academy at which they were elected or during which the terms of their predecessors expired and shall serve until the close of the succeeding Annual Meeting.

SECTION 4. ELECTION OR AUTOMATIC SUCCESSION TO OFFICE.

A. **President, President Elect and Immediate Past President.** The President Elect shall succeed to the office of President and the Vice President shall succeed to the office of President Elect without further election upon the expiration of the terms of the persons occupying those offices. Upon expiration of his term, the President shall be considered the Immediate Past President for a period of one year.

B. **Vice President, Secretary and Treasurer.** The Vice President, Secretary and Treasurer shall be elected by the voting members of the Academy of mail ballot. By no later than February 1st of each year the Committee on Nominations shall meet and submit to the Executive Director a list of candidates for each such office. The procedure for the nomination of additional candidates by petition and the election by mail ballot set forth in Chapter II, Section 7 shall apply.

SECTION 5. VACANCIES:

A. President. In the event the office of President becomes vacant, the President Elect shall serve as President for the unexpired term, in addition to serving a full term in that office in his own right.

B. President Elect. In the event the office of President Elect becomes vacant, the Vice President shall serve as President Elect for the unexpired term in addition to serving a full term in that office in his own right.

C. Vice President. In the event in the office of Vice President becomes vacant, the Secretary shall assumes the functions of the Vice President for the unexpired portion of the term in addition to his other duties. A new President Elect for the following year shall then be elected by mail ballot in accordance with the procedure described in Section 4B.

D. Secretary. In the event the office of Secretary becomes vacant, the President shall appoint a successor pro tem to serve until a new Secretary can be elected in accordance with the procedure described in Section 4B.

E. Treasurer. In the event the office of Treasurer becomes vacant, the President shall appoint a successor pro tem to serve until the next meeting of the General Assembly when a successor shall be elected.

F. Immediate Past President. In the event the office of Immediate Past President becomes vacant, no successor shall be appointed but the President shall assume the duties of the vacated office.

SECTION 6. RECALL:

Any Elected Officer of the Academy may be recalled as provided in the Procedures for Recall of District Executive Council Members and Elected Officers incorporated herein by reference.

CHAPTER VIII - APPOINTIVE OFFICERS

SECTION 1. DESIGNATIONS:

The Appointive Officers of the Academy shall consist of an Executive Director, an Editor (or Co-Editors) of the official publications of the Academy and such other positions as the Executive Council may from time to time determine.

SECTION 2. DUTIES:

A. Executive Director. The Executive Director shall administer the facilities and staff of the Academy under the direction and supervision of the President and the Executive Council and shall perform such other duties as they may assign to him.

B. Editor. The Editor (or Co-Editors) of the official publications shall exercise full editorial control thereover, subject only to the policies established by the Executive Council and the General Assembly.

C. Other Appointive Officers. Other Appointive Officers shall perform such duties as the President and Executive Council may prescribe.

SECTION 3. APPOINTMENT AND TERM OF OFFICE:

All Appointive Officers shall be appointed by the Executive Council for one-year terms, except for the Editor (or Co-Editors) who shall serve for three years.

SECTION 4. VACANCY:

In the event of a vacancy in the office of the Editor (or Co-Editors) the Executive Council shall appoint a successor for the unexpired term or for a full term of three years.

CHAPTER IX - FEES, DUES AND FISCAL MATTERS

SECTION 1. FISCAL YEAR:

The fiscal year of the Academy shall be from January 1 to December 31.

SECTION 2. FEES AND DUES:

A. General. Initiation fees shall be paid within 30 days after receipt of the invitation to join the Academy. (See Chapter I, Section 4.) Members who are reclassified shall pay any difference in initiation fees between the old and the new membership categories except Student Members who do not pay an initiation fee upon reclassification into another membership category. (See Chapter I, Section 8.) Annual dues are due on January 1. Members whose dues are not received by March 1 shall be assessed a $50 penalty. If the dues and any applicable penalty have not been received by May 1, membership will automatically be terminated. (See Chapter I, Section II).

B. Petitions for Waiver of Fees, Dues or Other Financial Obligations. The Executive Council shall have the power to reduce or waive a member's payment of fees, dues or other financial obligations for good cause shown by petition submitted to the Secretary.

C. Amounts. The amounts of fees and dues payable by the various categories of members of the Academy are as follows

Membership Classification	Initiation Fee	Annual Dues
1. Active Members	$200	$ 375
2. Associate Members	$150	$ 140
3. Academic Members	$ 50	$ 125
4. Student Members	None	$ 50
5. Nonresident Members	$ 50	$ 125
6. Retired Members	None	$ 35
7. Life Members	None	None
8. Honorary Members	None	None

Life and Retired Members shall pay for a subscription to the official journal, if one is desired. No additional payment shall be required for such a subscription for the other membership classifications.

SECTION 3. SPECIAL ASSESSMENTS:

In order to meet expenses of an unforeseen or nonreocurring nature the General Assembly may from time to time approve the imposition of a special assessment on all or part of the dues-paying membership of the Academy. Any such assessment shall be approved by a two-thirds majority of the members present and voting at the Annual Meeting of the General Assembly or at a special meeting called for that purpose. The assessment shall be payable by the members of such districts and such classifications of dues-paying members and in such a manner as the General Assembly may determine.

SECTION 4. FUNDS AND PROPERTY:

A. General. All funds and property received by the Academy through dues, fees, gifts, bequests or otherwise shall be utilized only to further the purposes of the Academy. The administration of the Grace Rogers Spalding Journal Endowment Fund for the support of the Academy's official publications, of the Memorial Fund for student loans and scholarships and for other charitable and educational projects to promote the objectives of the Academy, and of all other funds belonging to the Academy is vested in the Executive Council.

B. Safeguarding and Investment of Funds. The Treasurer shall authorize the deposit or investment of the funds of the Academy in such accounts, certificates of deposit, money market funds, commercial paper, stocks, bonds or other securities as he may deem appropriate under guidelines which shall be established by the Executive Council. The

Council may authorize the employment of such investment advisors, corporate custodians and auditors as it deems appropriate in connection with the investment and safekeeping of such funds. The Council may authorize the commingling of part or all of the various funds administered by the Council (including endowment and memorial funds) in a single investment fund, provided that adequate records are maintained to show at all times the proportionate shares (both principal and income) of each such fund in the commingled fund.

C. Signature Authority. All bills, notes, checks and other instruments for the payment of money and all stock certificates, bonds and other securities shall be signed or countersigned by such Elective or Appointive Officers and in such manner as shall from time to time be prescribed by the Executive Council.

SECTION 5. BORROWINGS AND MORTGAGES:

The Academy shall have the power to borrow money for its corporate purposes at such rates of interest as the Executive Council may determine without regard to the restrictions of any usury law; to issue notes, bonds, and other obligations; and to secure any of its obligations by mortgage, pledge or deed of trust of all or any of its property, franchises and income; all as may from time to time be deemed appropriate by the Executive Council.

CHAPTER X - AMERICAN BOARD OF PERIODONTOLOGY

SECTION 1. NAME AND PURPOSE:

The Academy shall sponsor the American Board of Periodontology (hereinafter referred to as the "Board") whose purpose shall be to elevate standards of periodontic practice by examining the qualifications and competence of dentists who voluntarily apply to the Board for certification as diplomates.

SECTION 2. DUTIES:

The Board shall examine candidates for designation as diplomates of the American Board of Periodontology. The activities of the Board shall conform to the requirements of the Council on Dental Education of the American Dental Association applicable to specialty boards in dentistry. The Board shall make an annual report to the Executive Council and the General Assembly.

SECTION 3. COMPOSITION:

The Board shall be composed of eight Active Members who are diplomates of the Board. Members of the Board shall serve for staggered six-year terms. No person may serve as a member of the Board for more than one term.

SECTION 4. NOMINATIONS:

A. Nominating Committee. The Nominating Committee for the American Board of Periodontology shall consist of one Active Member from each of the eight districts, to be elected as set forth in Chapter VI, Section 9. Members of the Nominating Committee shall serve staggered three-year terms. No person may serve more than two consecutive terms and candidates for District Council seats and members of the Executive Council shall not be eligible to serve on the Nominating Committee. The chairmanship of the Nominating Committee shall be rotated annually among the eight District members according to the numerical sequence of the Districts set forth in Chapter VI, Section 2.

B. Nominating Procedure. By no later than February 1st of each year the Nominating Committee for the Board shall meet and submit to the Executive Director a list containing the names of at least two candidates for each seat on the Board which will become vacant during that year. Additional candidates may be nominated by petition in accordance with the procedure described in Chapter II, Section 7.

SECTION 5. ELECTION:

The Directors of the American Board of Periodontology shall be elected by mail ballot sent to all voting members of the Academy. The election procedure shall be governed by the provisions set forth in Chapter II, Section 7.

CHAPTER XI - OFFICIAL PUBLICATION

SECTION 1: NAME AND FREQUENCY:

The official publication of the Academy shall be *The Journal of Periodontology*, which shall be published at least quarterly.

SECTION 2. OBJECT

The object of the official publication shall be to report, chronicle and evaluate matters of scientific and professional interest with particular emphasis on those activities as they relate to periodontology.

SECTION 3. SUBSCRIPTION RATE.

The Executive Council shall determine the subscription rate.

SECTION 4. CONTROL.

Ultimate control over the official publication shall be vested in the Executive Council. The Editor shall have full control over editorial matters, subject only to the policies established by the Executive Council and the General Assembly.

CHAPTER XII - ORGANIZATION OF THE ANNUAL MEETING

SECTION 1. GENERAL:

The Annual Meeting of the Academy shall be organized by the Committee on the Annual Meeting. The chairman of that Committee shall serve as the Director of the Annual Meeting and shall have primary responsibility for the organization of the Annual Meeting. The Director shall be guided by the Manual on Annual Meetings promulgated by the Executive Council, which shall have ultimate responsibility for approval of the plans made by the Director and the Committee on the Annual Meeting.

SECTION 2. SCIENTIFIC SESSIONS:

The Academy shall hold scientific sessions for the purpose of disseminating knowledge and improving the professional skills of the members of the Academy. Annual scientific sessions shall be held in conjunction with the Annual Meeting of the Academy at such time and place as the Executive Council may determine. The Executive Council may approve the organization of additional scientific sessions at other times during the year.

CHAPTER XIII - DISCIPLINARY PROCEDURES

SECTION 1. PROFESSIONAL CONDUCT:

The professional conduct of the members of this Academy shall be governed by the *Principles of Ethics and Code of Professional Conduct* of the American Dental Association; provided, however, that for nonresidents of the United States the ethical principles of the member's recognized national dental association shall supersede said *Principles* in cases of conflict.

SECTION 2. CONDUCT SUBJECT TO DISCIPLINE:

A member may be subject to disciplinary sanctions if he is found to have:

(a) committed a felony;

(b) violated the dental practice act of the state or province in which he practices; or

(c) violated the *Principles of Ethics* or other ethical principles applicable under Chapter XIII, Section 1.

SECTION 3. DISCIPLINARY SANCTIONS:

Members found to have engaged in conduct subject to discipline may be placed under a sentence of censure, suspension from membership or termination of membership depending on the gravity of that conduct.

A. Censure. A sentence of censure is an official reprimand by the Academy imposed for minor instances of misconduct. No loss of membership privileges in involved.

B. Suspension. See Chapter I, Section 10. A sentence of suspension from membership may be imposed for misconduct of a more serious nature.

C. Termination. See Chapter I, Section 11. A sentence terminating a member's membership may only be imposed in cased involving misconduct of the gravest nature.

SECTION 4. DISCIPLINARY PROCEEDINGS.

A. Preliminary Investigation. Instances of sanctionable conduct by members of the Academy shall be reported to the chairman of the Committee on Ethics, who shall either himself or through a designated representative conduct a preliminary factual investigation. The chairman will then call a meeting of the full committee which shall determine whether or not to recommend to the Executive Council that a hearing be held.

B. Hearing. If the Executive Council approves the recommendation of the Committee on Ethics that a hearing be held, it shall direct the Secretary of the Academy to send a written notice to the accused member by certified mail at least 60 days prior to the date of the hearing setting forth the time and place of the hearing and describing the member's alleged misconduct. The Council shall appoint a special committee to serve as the hearing body. The special committee shall consist of three members of the Executive Council and shall elect its own chairman. The accused shall have the right of determining whether or not the hearing will be open to other members of the Academy.

At the hearing the accused will be given the opportunity to present his defense to all charges brought against him. He may present his defense *pro se*, or may choose to be represented by another member of the Academy or by legal counsel of his choice at his expense. The accused shall also have the right to arrange at his own expense for a court reporter to make a transcription of the hearing.

After reviewing all of the evidence the special committee shall make detailed findings of fact and shall determine what sanction should be imposed, if any. A copy of the committee's decision and a notice informing the accused of his right to appeal shall be sent by the Secretary of the Academy to the accused by certified mail within ten days of the decision. Copies of the decision shall also be furnished to the chairmen of the Committee on Ethics and the Executive Council. The decision shall not become effective until the end of the thirty day period for taking an appeal therefrom, or in the event that an appeal has been filed, until the appeal is resolved.

C. Appeal to the Executive Council. If the decision of the special committee has resulted in the imposition of a sanction, the accused may appeal the decision to the Executive Council by filing a notice of appeal with the Secretary of the Academy within 30 days after the decision. Within 60 days after the date of the decision the accused shall submit to the Secretary a written memorandum setting forth his grounds for appeal. The Secretary shall have 30 days after the receipt of the accused's memorandum to file a response thereto. Additional briefs may be filed by the accused, the special committee or the person who originated the complaint against the accused within 120 days after the date of the decision.

The Executive Council shall then conduct a hearing on the accused's appeal, but without the participation of any member of the Council who served on the special committee. The Council shall be provided with copies of all memoranda, briefs, and the decision and record from the hearing of the special committee (including any available transcript of the proceedings and copies of all evidence reviewed by the committee). A notice setting forth the time and place of the hearing on appeal shall be sent to the accused by certified mail at least 30 days prior to the date of the hearing, with a copy to the chairman of the Committee on Ethics.

After reviewing all of the evidence the Executive Council shall issue a written opinion setting forth its decision on the appeal and its reasons therefore. The Council shall have the power to: (a) dismiss the appeal as being untimely if the notice of appeal was not filed within the deadlines established above; (b) remand the case of the special committee if it finds that the accused was not afforded all the procedural rights due to him under these Bylaws; (c) uphold the decision of the special committee and the sanction imposed; (d) reverse the decision of the special committee, thereby exonerating the accused; or (e) remand the case to the special committee with instructions to impose a lesser sanction. A copy of the decision of the Executive Council shall be sent to the accused by certified mail within ten days and to the chairman of the special committee and the Committee on Ethics.

CHAPTER XIV - ORGANIZATION OF POSTDOCTORAL PROGRAM DIRECTORS

SECTION 1. NAME:

The Academy shall sponsor the Organization of Postodoctoral Program Directors (hereinafter the "Organization".)

SECTION 2. MEMBERSHIP.

Membership in the Organization shall be open to all directors of postdoctoral programs in periodontology.

SECTION 3. CHAIRMAN:

The Organization shall select a chairman from among its members, who shall serve a maximum of three years.

SECTION 4. MEETINGS:

The Organization shall meet annually at the time of Annual Meeting of the Academy. The chairman shall prepare and circulate on agenda to the members of the Organization prior to the meeting.

SECTION 5. PURPOSE AND DUTIES:

The purpose and duties of the Organization shall include the following:

(a) To prepare a Registry of approved and provisionally approved programs in periodontology, and make the registry available to all institutions of dental education and all prospective postdoctral students at their request.

(b) To assist Committee on Membership of the Academy in obtaining Student Members.

(c) To make available to the Executive Director of the Academy complete lists of those who have successfully completed their postdoctoral program.

(d) To maintain a list of students accepted for postdoctoral programs and make it available to program directions and the Executive Director of the Academy.

(e) To maintain a list of qualified applicants who have bee rejected by a program because of lack of space, and make it available to program directions and the Executive Director of the Academy.

(f) To maintain a list of educators in periodontology who are seeking academic employment and make the list available to any dental education institution upon request.

CHAPTER XV - MISCELLANEOUS

SECTION 1. AMENDMENTS:

These Bylaws may be amended at any meeting of the General Assembly at which a quorum is present by a two-thirds vote of the members present and voting; provided that a description of the proposed Amendments shall have been included in the notice of such meeting.

SECTION 2. REGISTERED OFFICE:

The registered office of the Academy shall be at such place as the Executive Council may from time to time determine.

SECTION 3. BOOKS AND RECORDS:

The following books and records shall be kept at a place designated by the Executive Council (a) books and records of account; (b) minutes of the meetings of the General Assembly and the Executive Council; (c) reports of committees, foundations and other bodies of the Academy; (d) a current list of the members of the Executive Council and the officers of the Academy together with their business addresses; and (e) a roster of a voting members of the Academy by district.

SECTION 4. INSPECTION OF BOOKS AND RECORDS:

Any member of record of the Academy for at least six months immediately preceding his demand shall have the right upon at least 10 days' written demand to examine in person or by agent or attorney, during usual business hours, the minutes of meetings of the Executive Council and the General Assembly and the list of members of the Academy, and to make extracts therefrom.

An inspection authorized by this Section may be denied to such member or other person upon his refusal to furnish to the Academy an affidavit that such inspection will not be used for a purpose which is in the interest of a business or object other than the best interest of the Academy.

SECTION 5. INDEMNIFICATION:

The Academy shall indemnify each employee and volunteer who participates in any of its committees or programs against liability and expenses, including attorney's fees, incurred in connection with any legal action in which the volunteer or employee is made a defendant by reason of the volunteer or employee's good faith efforts on behalf of the Academy. This indemnification does not extend to conduct undertaken by a volunteer or employee in bad faith, in violation of law, or contrary to any rule or policy of the Academy or a committee. As a condition of receiving indemnification, the volunteer or employee shall allow the Academy to appoint counsel for him or her and shall agree to a coordinated defense to the extent deemed appropriate by the Academy. Counsel appointed for the volunteer or employee may be the same as counsel appointed to represent the Academy and/or other volunteers or employees.

SECTION 6. GENDER AND NUMBER:

All nouns, pronouns and any variations thereof shall be deemed to refer to the masculine, feminine, singular and plural as the identity of the person or persons may require.

SECTION 7. HEADINGS:

Article and Section titles and captions contained in these Bylaws are inserted only as a convenience and for reference, and in no way define, limit or extend the intent of any provision hereof.

Appendix C
Annual Meetings of The American Academy of Periodontology

Please note that dates were not available for all meetings; this information is included when possible.

1914
November 5-7
Willard Hotel
Washington DC

1915
September 20-22
Statler Hotel
Detroit, Michigan

1916
July 20-22
Pittsburgh, Pennsylvania

1917
New York, New York

1918
Chicago, Illinois

1919
New Orleans, Louisiana

1920
Boston, Massachusetts

1921
New York, New York

1922
Cincinnati, Ohio

1923
Cleveland, Ohio

1924
Atlanta, Georgia

1925
Louisville, Kentucky

1926
New York, New York

1927
Detroit, Michigan

1928
Minneapolis, Minnesota

1929
Washington, DC

1930
Colorado Springs, Colorado

1931
Memphis, Tennessee

1932
Buffalo, New York

1933
Chicago, Illinois

1934
St. Paul, Minnesota

1935
New Orleans, Louisiana

1936
San Francisco, California

1937
Atlantic City, New Jersey

1938
St. Louis, Missouri

1939
Milwaukee, Wisconsin

1940
Cleveland, Ohio

1941
Houston, Texas

1942
no meeting held

1943
Chicago, Illinois

1944
no meeting held

1945
no meeting held

1946
October 17-19
Birmingham, Alabama

1947
July 31- August 2
Boston, Massachusetts

1948
September 9-11
Chicago, Illinois

1949
October 13-15
San Francisco, California

1950
October 26-28
Atlantic City, New Jersey

1951
October 11-13
Washington DC

1952
September 4-6
St. Louis, Missouri

1953
September 24-26
Cleveland, Ohio

1954
November 4-6
Miami Beach, Florida

1955
October 13-15
Sheraton Palace Hotel
San Francisco, California

1956
September 27-29
Claridge Hotel
Atlantic City, New Jersey

1957
October 31-November 2
Di Lido Hotel
Miami Beach, Florida

1958
November 6-8
Baker Hotel
Dallas, Texas

1959
September 10-12
Barbizon-Plaza Hotel
New York, New York

1960
October 13-15
Miramar Hotel
Santa Monica, California

1961
October 20-25
departing from Philadelphia, Pennsylvania on board the M.S. Bergensfjord enroute to Burmuda

1962
October 25-27
Carillon Hotel
Miami Beach, Florida

1963
October 9-12
New York Hilton Hotel
New York, New York

1964
November 4-7
Sheraton Palace Hotel
San Francisco, California

1965
November 3-6
Dunes Hotel
Las Vegas, Nevada

1966
November 9-12
St. Anthony Hotel
San Antonio, Texas

1967
October 25-28
Mayflower Hotel
Washington, DC

1968
October 23-26
The Diplomat Hotel
Hollywood, FL

1969
October 8-11
Benjamin Franklin Hotel
Philadelphia, Pennsylvania

1970
September 16-19
Hotel Bonaventure
Montreal, Quebec

1971
October 6-9
Sherman House
Chicago, Illinois

1972
October 25-28
Town and Country Hotel
San Diego, California

1973
October 24-27
Convention Center
San Antonio, Texas

1974
October 2-5
Regency Hyatt Hotel
Atlanta, Georgia

1975
September 24-27
Radison Hotel
Minneapolis, Minnesota

1976
November, 17-20
San Francisco Hilton
San Francisco, California

1977
October 5-8
Sheraton Boston Hotel
Boston, Massachusetts

1978
September 27-30
Phoenix Civic Center
Phoenix, Arizona

1979
October 31-November 3
Seattle Center
Seattle, Washington

1980
October 8-11
Stouffer's Riverfront Towers
St. Louis, Missouri

1981
October 21-24
The Sheraton Centre
Toronto, Ontario

1982
October 6-9
Disneyland Hotel
Anaheim, California

1983
September 28-October 1
Atlanta Hilton
Atlanta, Georgia

1984
September 19-22
New Orleans Hilton Hotel
New Orleans, Louisiana

1985
September 11-14
San Francisco Hilton & Tower
San Francisco, California

1986
September 24-27
Stouffer Inn on the Square
Cleveland, Ohio

1987
October 21-24
Hyatt Regency/Marriott City
Center Hotels
Denver, Colorado

1988
October 26-29
Sheraton Harbor Island Hotels
San Diego, California

1989
October 25-28
Sheraton Washington Hotel
Washington, DC

Appendix D
Diplomates
The American
Board of Periodontology

Abrams, Herbert
Abrams, Irving
Adams, Donald F.
Adams, Frank L.
Adcock, John E.
Ahl, Dennis R.
Alderman, Norman E.
Alexander, Perry C.
Alford, Leroy B.
Algus, Seymour
Allen, Andrew L.
Allen, William R.
Alloy, Jack
Amano, Donald S.
Ambrose, James A.
Ambrose, John M.
Ammons, William F.
Antonini, Charles J.
Antoon, James W.
Apfelbaum, Steven D.
Ariaudo, Arnold A.
Armistead, R. Lewis
Arnett, Roy L.
Arnold, Ralph M.
Arvins, Allan N.
Asato, Herbert M.
Asnis, Saul Baxt
Assad, Daniel A.
Austin, Grace B.
Awrach, Murry A.
Baer, Paul N.
Bahat, Oded
Baima, Robert F.
Ball, Edward L, Jr.
Barr, Charles E.
Barrington, Erwin P.
Barton, Nancy S.
Beach, Matthew M.
Becker, Burton E.
Becker, Robert
Becker, William
Bell, W. Bernard
Belting, Charles M.
Benjamin, Sheldon D.
Bentman, J.J.
Bergquist, John J.
Berman, Charles L.
Bernbach, Alan L.
Beube, Frank E.
Bier, Sanford J.
Blacharsh, Carl
Blades, Duncan
Blank, Robert D.
Bleier, Larry P.
Block, Philip Lloyd
Bloom, Jack
Booker, Brooks W.
Boscarino, Joseph J.
Bosworth, Bruce L.
Bowen, Richard P.
Bowers, Gerald M.
Bral, Michael
Brasher, W. James
Brayshaw, Horace A.
Breault, Michael R.
Brenman, Henry S.
Brennan, William A.
Bressman, Edward
Bricken, Herbert
Britt, Michael R.
Broline, Leslie E.
Broome, William C.
Brown, Frederic H.
Brown, I. Stephen
Brownstein, Carol N.
Broxson, Alfred W.
Bruner, Hugh H., Jr.
Brunsvold, Michael A.
Buckwald, Howard
Bueltmann, Kenneth W.
Burman, Louis R.
Burnette, Elmer W., Jr.
Bye, Fred L.
Cacciatore, Angelo C.
Campana, Luis R.
Caplan, Philip S.
Cappetta, Emil G.
Cardinal, Stanley J.
Carroll, Peter B.
Carson, Robert E.
Cassingham, R. Jack
Caswell, Wallis D.
Caton, Jack G, Jr.
Caudill, Richard F.
Cederbaum, Alvin D.
Chace, Richard
Chace, Richard, Jr.
Chacker, Frederic M.
Chaikin, Bernard S.
Charbeneau, Thomas D.
Chasens, Abram I.
Chilton, Neal W.
Church, Lloyd F.
Ciancio, Sebastian G.
Clark, James W.
Coatoam, Gary W.
Coats, Gilbert F.
Cohen, Abram
Cohen, Charles I.
Cohen, D. Walter
Coker, Mack E.
Coleton, Stuart H.
Collings, C.K.
Collins, Peter Howard
Common, John
Conant, Julian R.
Conner, H. Dalton
Conroy, Charles W.
Conway, James C.
Coogler, Arthur C.
Cook, Gary G.
Corey, John B.
Corley, J. Monty
Corn, Herman
Cornick, Martin, H.
Cornish, Eleanore
Corsair, Alexander
Courant, Paul R.
Craemer, Timothy D.
Craig, James Adam
Crayle, Leonard J.
Croft, Lloyd K.
Crumley, Phillip J.
Cummings, Donald E.
Dail, Ray A.
Dannenbaum, R.M.
Davis, Robert K.
Dayoub, Michael B.
Dehaven, Harold A., Jr.
Del Vecchio, Ronald A.
Dello Russo, Nicholas M.
DeNucci, Donald J.
Detamore, Robert J.
Detsch, Steven Gorgas
Dickinson, Gary L.
Dickler, Elliott H.
Diem, Charles R.
DiFranco, Charles F.
DiGiacinto, James
Dix, Robert L.
Dober, Larry

Dobronte, Frank
Dolgin, David
Donnenfeld, O.W.
Doran, Edward J.
Doyle, Bernard J.
Drury, Gerald I.
Duello, George V.
Dummett, C.O.
Dunlap, Robert M.
Durso, Peter J.
Dwyer, Michael S.
Edwards, Richard C.
Eisenberg, Robert J.
Eisenstein, Ira L.
Ellinger, Harley A., Jr.
Elliott, Harold S.
Elliott, John E.
Engler, William O.
Epstein, Stuart R.
Eskow, Robert N.
Evans, Gerald H.
Evian, Cyril I.
Ewen, Sol J.
Ezis, Ilmar
Fabrizio, Francis J.
Fancher, James P.
Faner, Richard M.
Fauth, Gregory L.
Favaloro, John L.
Fedi, Peter F., Jr.
Feingold, Jeffrey P.
Feldman, Roy S.
Feldman, Sylvan
Felts, Charles B., III
Ferris, Geraldine M.
Ferris, Robert T.
Ficara, Anthony J.
Filipowicz, Francis J.
Finlayson, Richard S.
Fischer, George E.
Fisher, Emile T.
Florence, Michael J.
Flynn, Mitchell L.
Folson, Stephen A.
Foshager, Vernon D.
Foss, Calvin L.
Foulke, Clark N.
Fox, Lewis
Francis, John K.
Frantzis, Theodosios G.
Franzetti, Joseph J.
Freedman, Jeffrey
Friedman, Nathan
Frisch, Joe
Fritz, Michael E.
Frumker, Sanford C.
Fry, Hiram R.
Frydman, Albert
Fuller, Walter W.
Gage, Raymond W., II
Gallagher, J.W.
Gallagher, Steven J.
Gardner, William M.
Gargiulo, Alphonse V.
Gargiulo, Anthony W.
Garnick, Jerry
Gartner, Richard R., Jr.
Gaston, David L.
Gelb, David A.
Geraci, Timothy F.
Gher, Marlin E., Jr.
Gian-Grasso, Joseph E.
Gillette, William B.
Gilmore, Earl
Gold, Arthur
Gold, Steven I.
Goldberg, Maurice
Goldhaber, Paul
Goldman, Henry M.
Goldstein, Avrum R.
Golomb, Ida M.
Gomer, Ronald M.
Goodman, Stephen F.
Goodstein, Fred
Gordon, Mark R.
Gottehrer, Neil R.
Gottsegen, Robert
Graham, Charles J.
Grant, Daniel A.
Gray, Jonathan L.
Gray, Ralph C.
Greco, George W.
Green, Barry L.
Green, Louis H.
Greene, Alan H.
Griffel, Alan S.
Griffin, L. Hill
Griffin, Terence J.
Groat, Jack E.
Grossman, Michael S.
Haddad, Abraham
Hagearty, Michael B.
Haggerty, Patrick C.
Hall, J. Richard
Hallmon, William W.
Halpern, Edward L.
Hamblen, Tolar N., Jr.
Hamilton, Jack N.
Hancock, Everett B.
Harless, Charles F.
Harrel, Stephen K.
Harrold, Charles Q.
Harvey, Brien V.
Hashim, James R.
Hattler, Arthur B.
Hawley, Charles E.
Hazen, Stanley P.
Hebert, Maurice R.
Heitman, Kenneth L.
Heller, Alvin W.
Henken, Eleanor C.
Henkin, Jeffrey M.
Hey, Ernest, G. A.
Hiatt, William H.
Hileman, Alvin C.
Hill, Roger W.
Hindman, Robert E.
Hine, Maynard K.
Hines, Richard A.
Hinrichs, James E.
Hirschfeld, Leonard S.
Hix, James O., III
Hoag, Philip M.
Hogan, Donald W.
Holen, Sheldon
Holmes, Corey H.
Holpuch, Russell L.
Horning, Gregory M.
Hoskins, Sam W., Jr.
Howell, Richard E.
Hughes, W.R.
Hurt, William C.
Hutchens, Luther H., Jr.
Hutchinson, Rowland A.
Hyde, Vernon E.
Iacono, Vincent J.
Ilchyshyn, Nicholas
Irons, Willis B.
Isenberg, Gerald A.
Israelson, Hilton
Ivancie, Gerald P.
Jaffin, Robert A.
Javed, Tariq
Jewson, Leonard G.
Jividen, Glenn J.
Johnson, Raymond E.
Johnson, Walter N.
Joondeph, Norman H.
Joseph, Charles E.
Julienne, Charles H.
Kakehasi, Samuel
Kaldahl, Wayne B.

Kalkwarf, Kenneth L.
Kaplowitz, Bernard M.
Karel, Irving A.
Kartman, Jules D.
Kassolis, James D.
Keagle, James G.
Keith, W. Kent
Kepic, Thomas J.
Killoy, William J.
Kirkland, George F., Jr.
Kirsch, Sanford
Kitzis, Stanley
Klassman, Barry
Klein, Robin
Kleinman, Preston R.
Klempert, Milton
Klingsberg, Jules
Kobrinksy, Samuel
Koch, Robert W.
Kohn, J. David
Kollar, John A., Jr.
Koteen, Seymour M.
Kramer, Gerald M.
Krauss, Richard S.
Kuhar, Kenneth J.
Laffitte, Herbert B.
Lainson, Phillip A.
Landman, Norman K.
Lane, James J.
Langer, Burton
Langford, L. Perry
Larato, Dominick C.
Lawrence, Joseph J.
Leabo, Walter
Legleu, John K.
Lekas, James S.
Levi, Paul A., Jr.
Levin, Martin A.
Levin, Marvin P.
Levin, Robert D.
Levine, Robert A.
Levine, Stephen D.
Levsky, Stanley S.
Levy, Leon
Levy, Paul K.
Lewis, A. Budner
Linz, Vincent A.
Lite, Theodore
Livingston, Herbert L.
Lobene, Ralph R.
Loewenthal, Bernard
Loftus, Edward R.
Lopp, Frederick B.
Loughlin, Dan M.
Lovelace, Bruce M.
Loving, Robert H.
Low, Samuel B.
Lubarr, Alan R.
Lubow, Richard M.
Lynch, Thomas J.
Lyon, Douglas R.
Lyons, Harry
Lytle, Floyd E.
Lytle, James D.
Mackler, Stephen
Madigan, James L.
Mahan, Charles J.
Mahon, Nicholas C.
Makins, Patrick C.
Malamed, Emanuel H.
Malinowski, Andrew S.
Malone, Frank J.
Manne, Marshall S.
Marinello, Richard F.
Marks, Manuel H.
Maupin, Clay C.
Maybury, Joseph E.
Mayhew, Donnie E.
Maynard, J. Gary, Jr.
Mazzella, Walter, J.
McDonald, Fred L.
McGuire, Michael K.
McKenzie, Gregg W.
McKenzie, John S.
McKenzie, William T.
McMullen, James A.
McNeely, Thomas E.
McQuade, Michael J.
Mecall, Richard A.
Meffert, Roland M.
Meitner, Sean W.
Mellonig, James T.
Meltzer, Alan M.
Michaelides, Paul L.
Miller, Edward F.
Miller, Garry M.
Miller, Richard L.
Mills, Michael P.
Mintz, Alan L.
Mishkin, Jack H.
Mitchell, Gerald A.
Montoya, Ralph G.
Moomaw, Robert C.
Moore, Timothy E.
Moore, Willa Y.
Morgan, William C., Jr.
Morgan, William J.
Moriarty, John D.
Morris, Melvin L.
Moser, Ernest H., Jr.
Moskow, Bernard S.
Moskowicz, Donald G.
Munk, Albert J.
Murphy, James L.
Nabers, Claude L.
Nabers, John M.
Nachazel, Delbert P.
Nakata, Ted M.
Neale, William S.
Nease, William J.
Neilson, John W.
Nevins, Myron
Newell, Donald H.
Newton, Dennis W., Jr.
Nosworthy, Donald G.
Novak, M. John
O'Bannon, James Y., Jr.
O'Leary, Tomothy J.
O'Neal, Robert B.
Ochsenbein, Clifford
Odrich, Ronald B.
Ogilvie, Alfred L.
Okun, Marvin N.
Older, Lester B.
Oliver, Richard C.
Oshrain, Herbert I.
Owings, James R., Jr.
Padgett, James L.
Palcanis, Kent G.
Parkel, Charles O., Jr.
Parsons, John C., Jr.
Patur, Benjamin
Paulsen, Albert G.
Peden, John W.
Pendergast, William J.
Perez-Febles, Joaquin
Peters, Jerome F.
Peterson, Ronald J.
Pfeifer, John S.
Phillips, Bradley L.
Pihlstrom, Bruce L.
Pizzurro, Robert E.
Plotzke, Anthony E.
Podlin, Bernard F.
Pollack, Ralph P.
Polson, Alan M.
Pomeranz, Melvin J.
Popper, Howard A.
Prichard, John F.

Prucha, Dan M.
Pruthi, Vijay K.
Quart, Arthur M.
Quintero, George
Radentz, William H.
Rainey, Bernard L.
Ralls, Stephen
Ramfjord, Sigurd
Rapley, John W.
Ratcliff, Perry A.
Rathofer, Steven A.
Raust, George T., Jr.
Rautiola, Clifton A.
Rees, Terry D.
Reeve, Charles M.
Reeves, Robert L.
Reeves, William G.
Reich, Gregory M.
Reiser, Gary M.
Reitan, Steven G.
Rethman, Michael P.
Ricchetti, Paul A.
Rice, Bruce H.
Rice, George W.
Rice, Steven N.
Richman, Colin S.
Rinck, Theodore, J.H.
Ritchey, Beryl T.
Robinson, Clyde M.
Robinson, James R.
Robinson, R. Earl
Rodden, Jeffrey W.
Roller, Neal W.
Romanow, Irving
Rose, Louis F.
Rosenberg, E.S.
Rosenberg, Marvin M.
Rosenberg, Ronald
Rosenberg, Sally
Rosenbluth, Morton
Rosenfeld, Alan L.
Rosenthal, S. Leonard
Rosner, David
Ross, Ira F.
Ross, James R.
Ross, Sheldon J.
Ross, Stanley E.
Rossmann, Jeffrey A.
Roth, Harry
Rothwell, Harry G., Jr.
Rott, Ronald R.
Rowan, Joseph E.

Rubelman, Peter A.
Ruben, Morris P.
Rubinoff, Craig H.
Ruggerio, Anthony C.
Saadoun, Andre P.
Saari, James T.
Sackler, Alvin M.
Samaha, Francis J.
Sanders, John J.
Sandifer, Johnny B.
Saunders, Kip W.
Savas, Athan
Schafer, Thomas J.
Schaffer, Erwin M.
Schallhorn, Robert G.
Scheffer, Miles H.
Scheidt, Michael J.
Schluger, Saul
Schoor, Robert S.
Schreiber, Harold R.
Schwartz, Murray
Schwartz, R. Stuart
Schwimer, David H.
Scopp, Irwin W.
Seibert, Jay S.
Seifert, John H.
Selipsky, Herbert
Senter, Alvin D.
Sepe, Walter W.
Shanbour, Gregory S.
Shannon, Thomas R.
Shapiro, Morton L.
Shapiro, Nathan
Shapoff, Cary A.
Sharaiha, Amal Z.
Sheridan, Phillip J.
Shick, Richard A.
Shields, Walter D.
Shields, Walton F.
Shiloah, Jacob
Shklar, Gerald
Shockett, Howard P.
Siegal, Don E.
Silberg, Mark E.
Silvers, Herbert F.
Simon, S. Lawrence
Simpson, David M.
Simring, Marvin
Singer, Richard J.
Singh, Surendra M.
Singletary, Macon M.
Smith, Randall L.

Smukler, Hyman
Snyder, Alvin J.
Sobkov, Theodore S.
Solomon, Marvin
Sonick, Michael K.
Sorensen, William P.
Spettel, W.R.
Staffileno, Harry, Jr.
Stahl, S. Sigmund
Staley, Barry B.
Stalker, William H.
Staub, Daniel M.
Stein, Stephen D.
Stepnick, Robert J.
Stern, Irving B.
Sternig, Martin
Sternlicht, Harold C.
Stewart, Geo. G.
Stillerman, Joseph J.
Stoller, Norman H.
Stoller, Stanley M.
Stolman, Joseph M.
Strong, Scott L.
Stuever, C.H., Jr.
Sugarman, Edward F.
Sugarman, Marvin M.
Sugarman, Richard
Suit, Stanley R.
Sullivan, John F.
Sumner, Charles F., III
Suzuki, Jon B.
Swan, Richard H.
Swenson, Henry M.
Tannenbaum, Paul
Tarnow, Dennis P.
Tavtigian, Richard
Telsey, Bernard
Tempel, Thomas R.
Thaller, Jack L.
Themann, William A.
Thomas, B.O.A.
Thomas, Lloyd G., Jr.
Thompson, Dennis M.
Tobias, James A.
Towle, Herbert J., III
Treado, Robert F.
Tress, Emanuel R.
Tuckman, Marvin A.
Tuffiash, Charles Mark
Turner, Alvin J.
Tyler, David C.
Uhrie, Ignatz G.

Ulrich, George
Umaki, Clyde S.
Uohara, George I.
Valentine, Randall L.
Vallins, Neal F.
Van Scotter, Donald E.
Van Swol, Ronald L.
Vanarsdall, Robert L. Jr.
Vandersall, David C.
Vaughan, Olin B.
Verino, Arthur R.
Versman, Kenneth J.
Vilardi, Mario A.
Vincent, Jack W.
Vogel, Richard I.
Wade, Byron M.
Wade, Curtis
Wagenberg, Barry D.
Waldrop, Thomas C.
Walker, Kahn K.
Wallace, A. Leigh
Warren, E.A.
Wasserman, Bernard
Watson, Walter J.
Weatherford, Thomas, II
Weiner, David E.
Weiner, Leonard
Weiss, Leon A.
Weiss, Richard C.
Welch, Robert D.
Wertheimer, F. W.
Wescott, Randall L.
Westbrook, James C., Jr.
Westbury, Lawrence W.
Wheeler, Philip V.
Whinston, George J.
Whitman, Jack K.
Wiebusch, F.B.
Wilkinson, Edward G.
Wilkinson, Raymond F.
Williams, Charles H.M.
Williams, Howard J.
Williams, John E., Jr.,
Wilson, Thomas G., Jr.
Winson, Dennis E.
Winter, Alan A.
Wirthlin, Milton R. Jr.
Withers, James A.
Witkin, George J.
Witte, E. Thompson
Wolfe, Barry
Wollman, Sheldon J.
Woodyard, Stephen G.
Yamada, Richard H.
Yudkoff, Irving
Yukna, Raymond A.
Zablotny, F.H.
Zakarin, Robert A.
Zaner, David J.
Zeren, Karl J.
Zingale, Joseph A.
Zupnik, Robert M.

Appendix E
Annual Meetings of the American Society of Periodontists

1962
July 5-7
Seattle, Washington

1963
May 5-8
Denver, Colorado

1964
May 18-20
Swampscott, Massachusetts

1965
May 10-12
Colorado Springs, Colorado

1966
May 19-21
Chicago, Illinois

1967
May 15-17
Colorado Springs, Colorado

Presidential Portraits. . . . .
a selection from the first 25 years

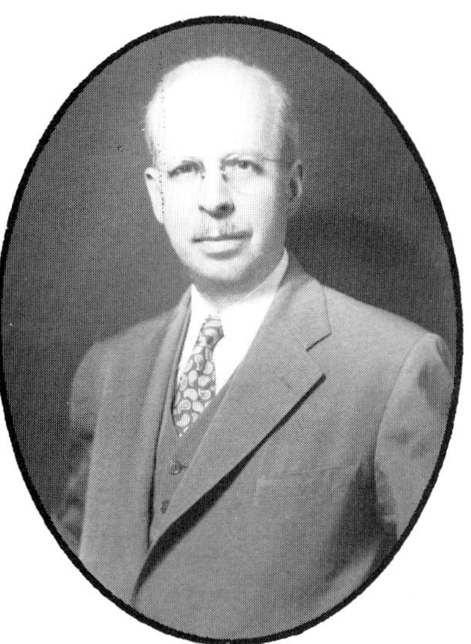

1917
John Oppie McCall*

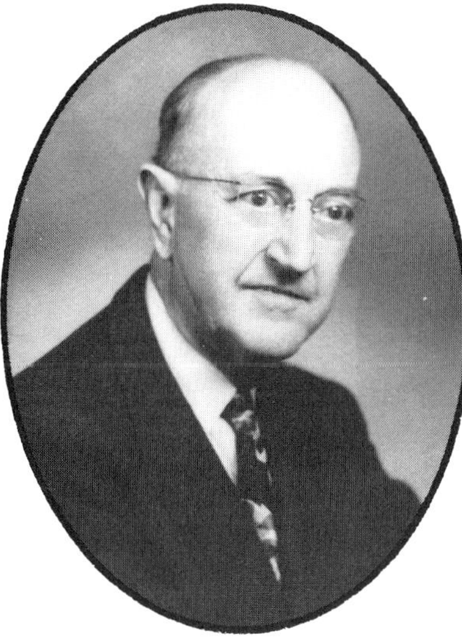

1928
Justin D. Towner*

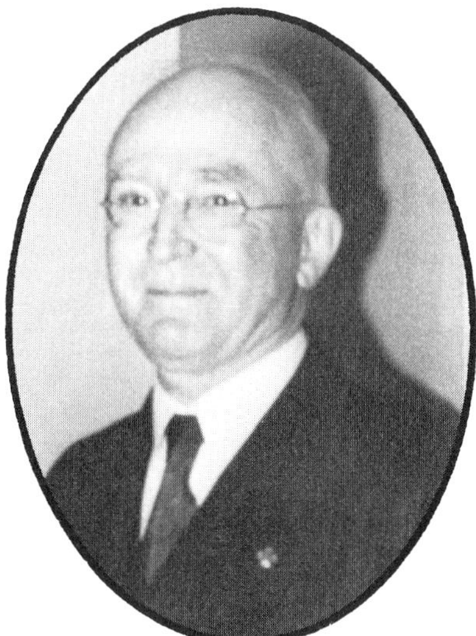

1925
Arthur H. Merritt*

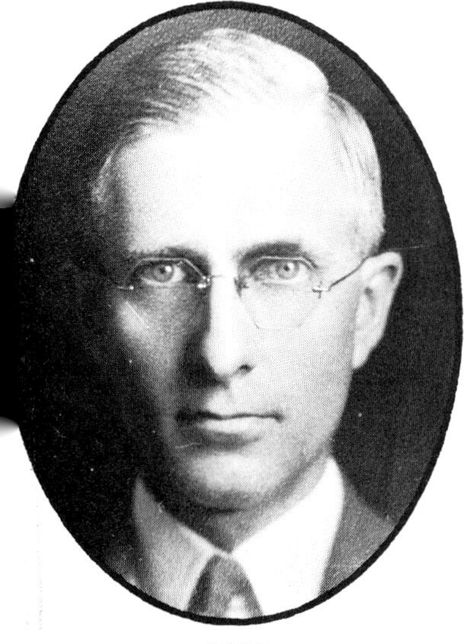

1932
Harold J. Leonard*

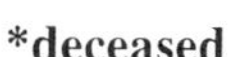

*deceased

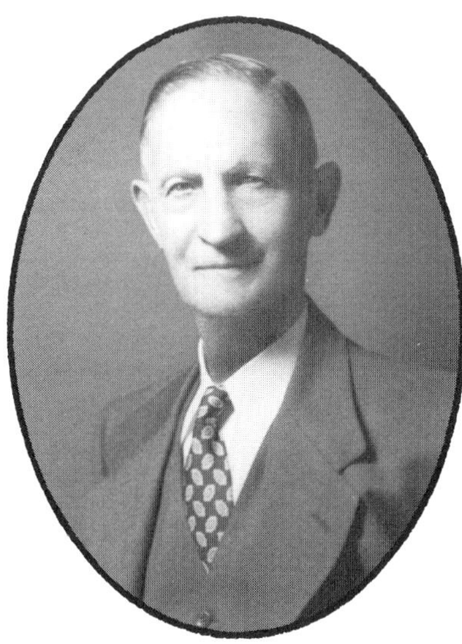

1937
Edward B. Spalding*

Presidents of the American Academy of Periodontology 1914 through 1989

Unfortunately, it was not possible to obtain photographs of all of the former presidents of the Academy. The previous page shows some of the Academy's early presidents, who are also included in this full chronological listing. Please note that photographs were drawn from the Academy archives and contributions by members of the Academy; therefore, not all photographs shown were taken during the presidental year.

An asterisk (*) indicates that the member is deceased.

1914, 1915
Austin F. James*

1916
Gillette Hayden*

1917
John Oppie McCall*

1918
J. Herbert Hood*

1919
Jules Sarrazin*

1920
Andrew J. McDonagh*

1921
Paul R. Stillman*

1922
Clyde M. Gearhart*

1923
Grace R. Spalding*

1924
Olin Kirkland*

1925
Arthur H. Merritt*

1926
M. Harry Garvin*

1927
Carlos H. Schott*

1928
Justin D. Towner*

1929
Julian Smith*

1930
Clyde C. Sherwood*

1931
Carl W. Hoffer*

1932
Harold J. Leonard*

1933
Benjamin Tishler*

1934
M. Monte Bettman*

1935
Walter H. Scherer*

1936
Haidee Weeks*

1937
Edward B. Spalding*

1938
Clayton H. Gracey*

1939
A. W. Bryan*

1940
Rudolph Kronfeld*
Thomas B. Hartzell*

1941
Isador Hirschfeld*

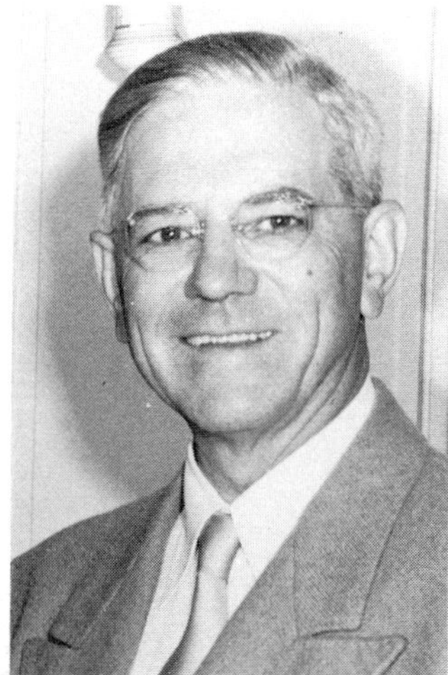

1942, 1943
Robert L. Dement*

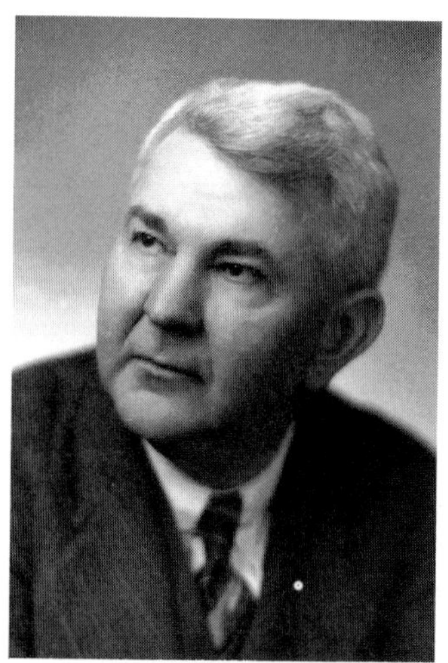

1944, 1945, 1946
Samuel R. Parks*

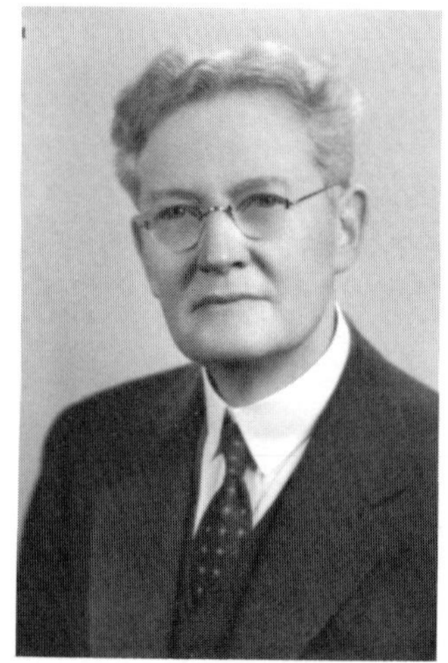

1947
Edgar D. Coolidge*

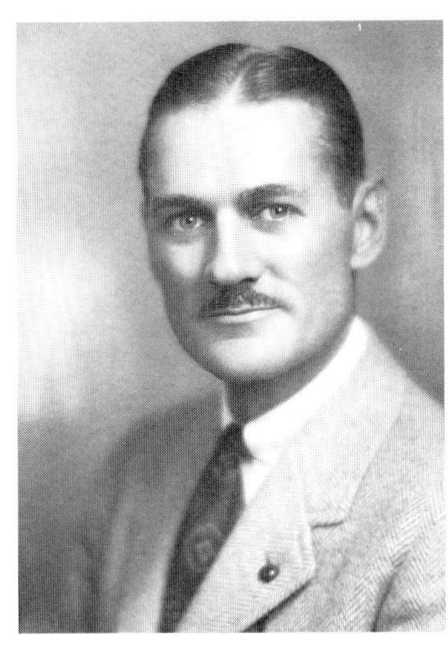

←
1948
Raymond E. Johnson

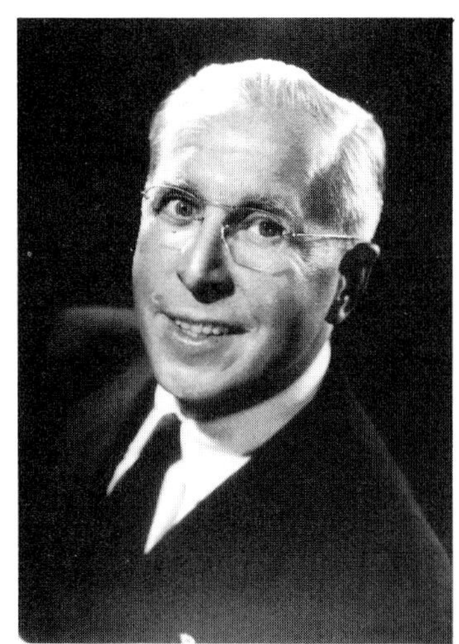

→
1949
Edward L. Ball*

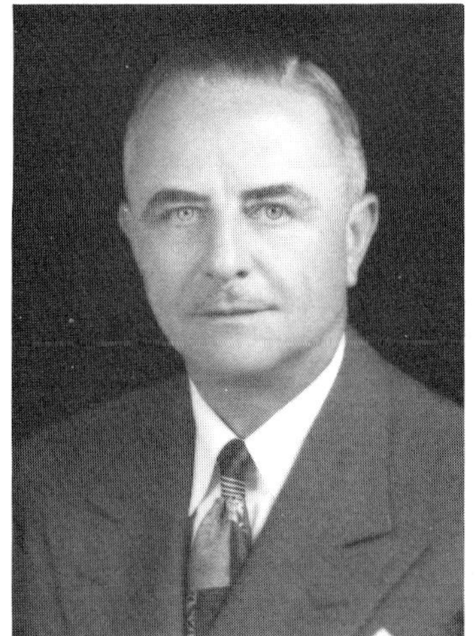

←
1950
Dickson G. Bell*

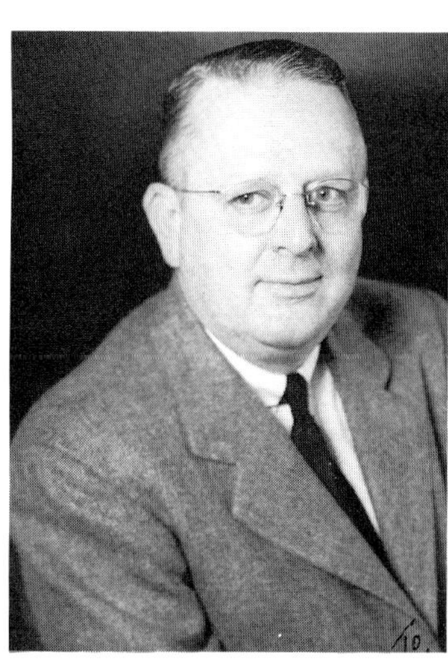

→
1951
Hunter S. Allen*

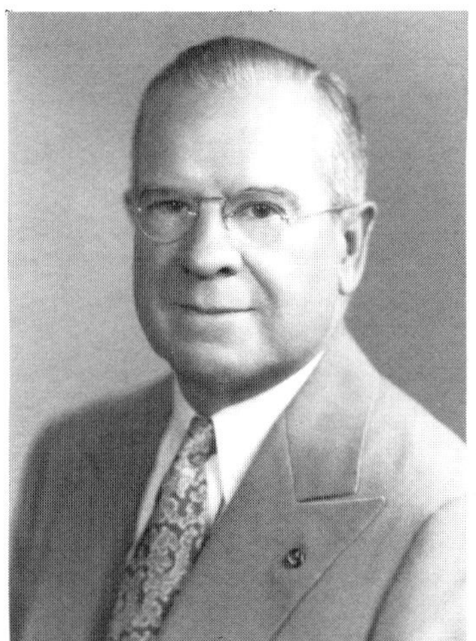

←
1952
James E. Aiguier*

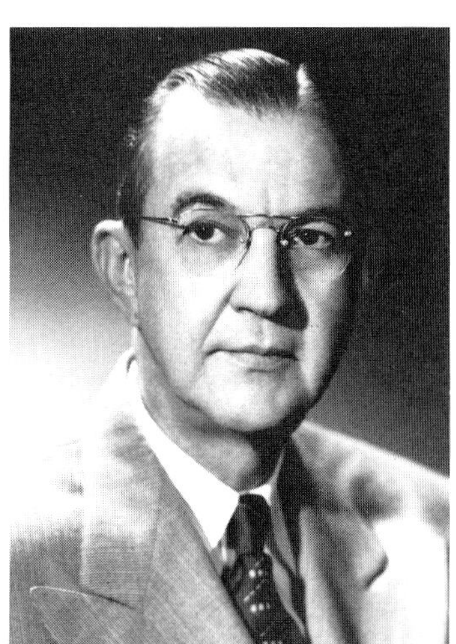

→
1953
Roy O. Elam*

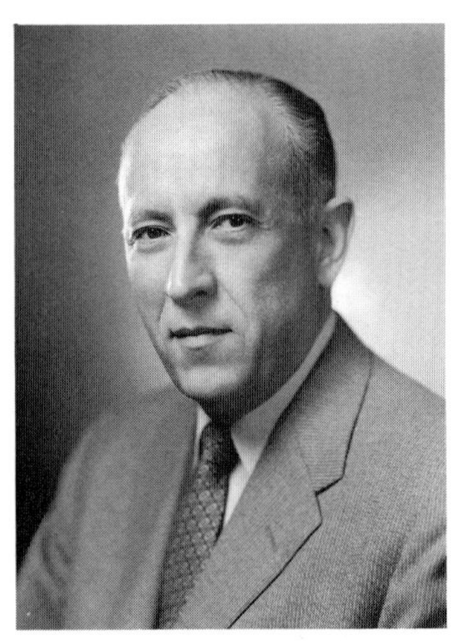

←

1954
Harry Lyons

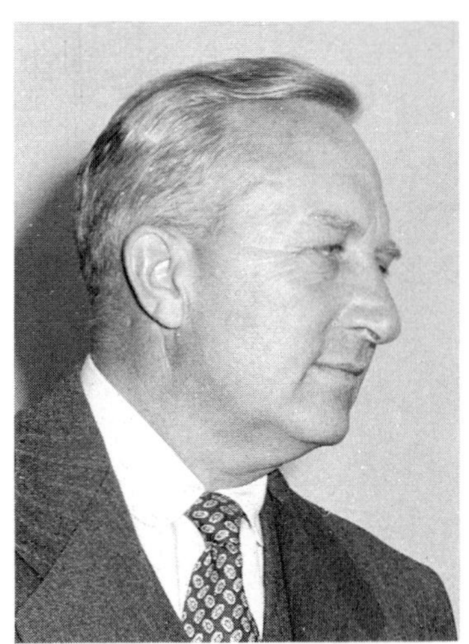

→

1955
Harold G. Ray*

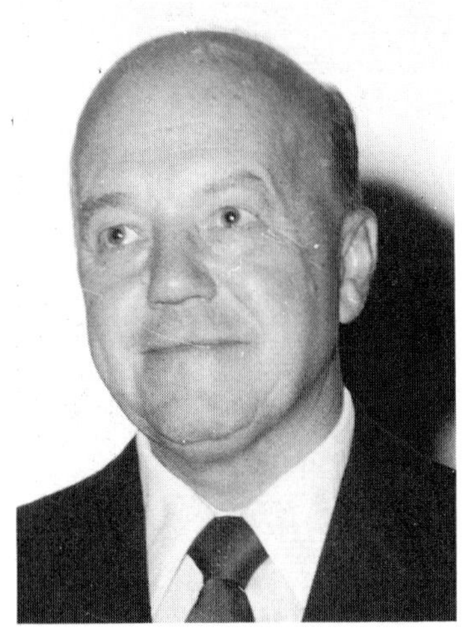

←

1956
Robert G. Kesel*

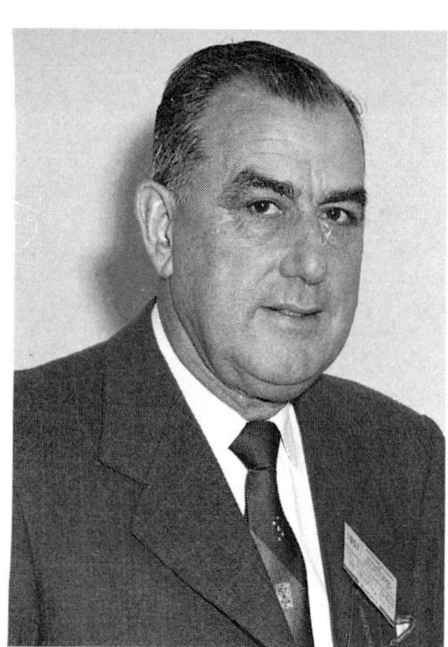

→

1957
Stanley C. Baker*

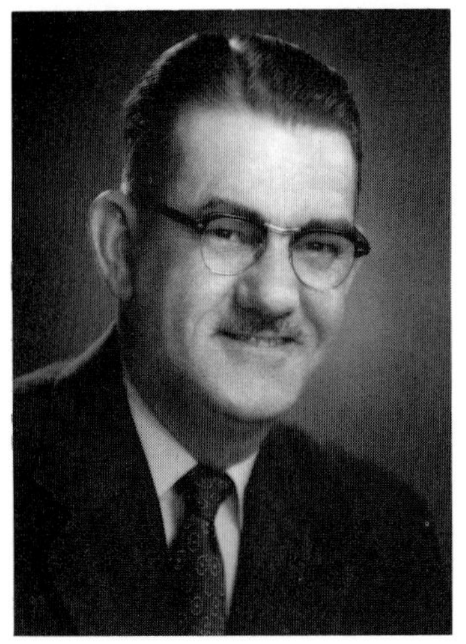

←

1958
Donald A. Kerr*

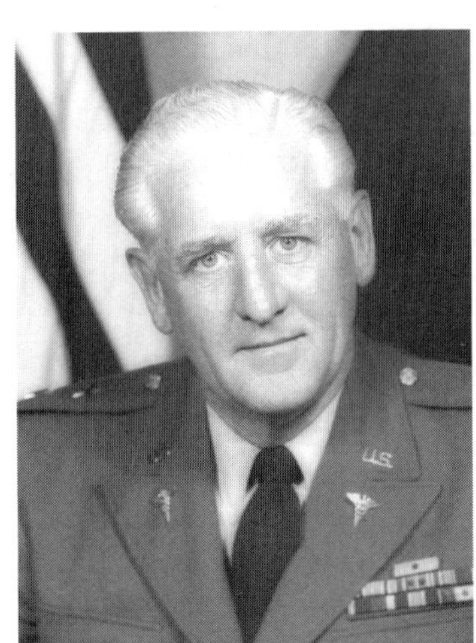

→

1959
Joseph L. Bernier*

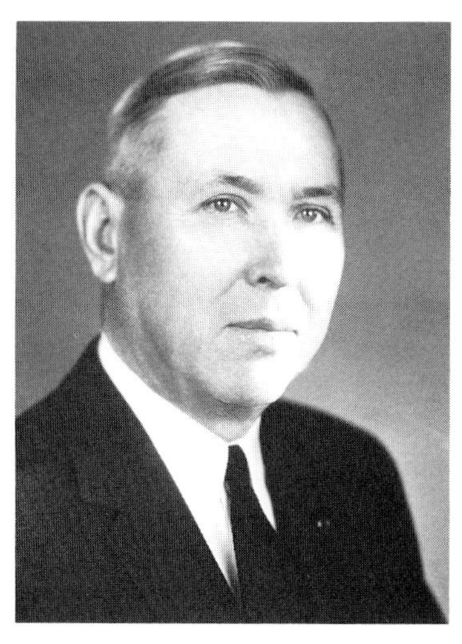

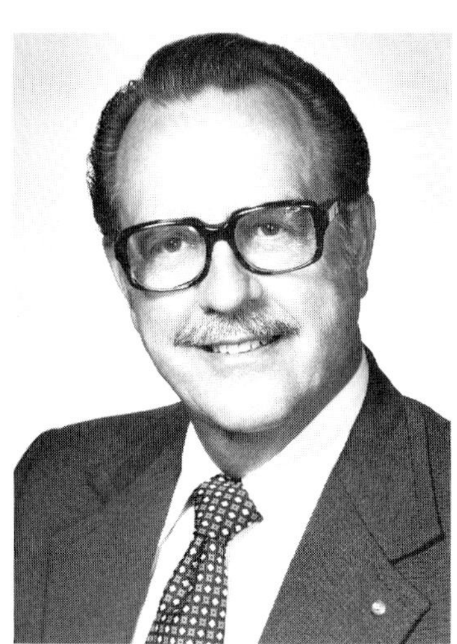

←
1960
James P. Hollers*

→
1961
B.O.A. Thomas

←
1962
Evert A. Archer*

→
1963
Sigurd P. Ramfjord

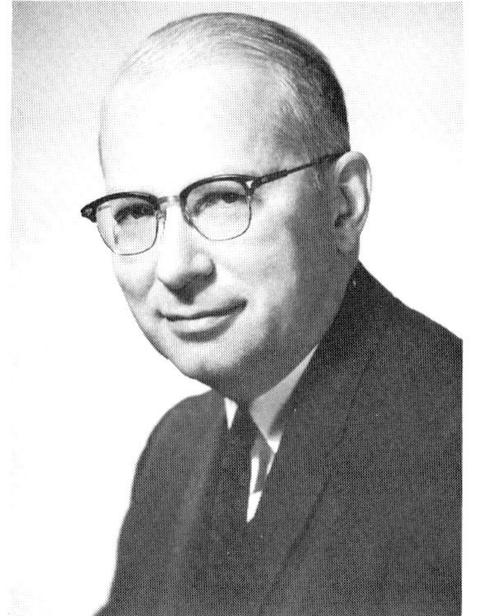

←
1964
Maynard K. Hine

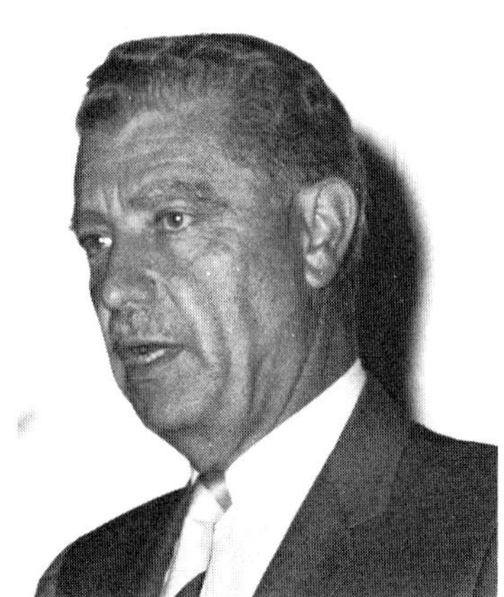

→
1965
Frank E. Beube

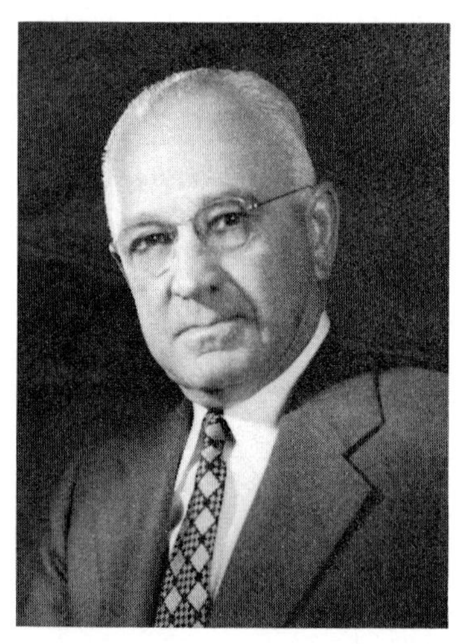

←
1966
Clarke E. Chamberlain*

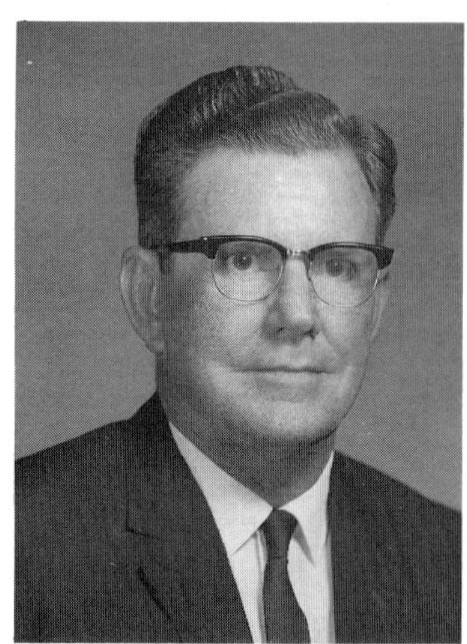

→
1967
John S. McKenzie*

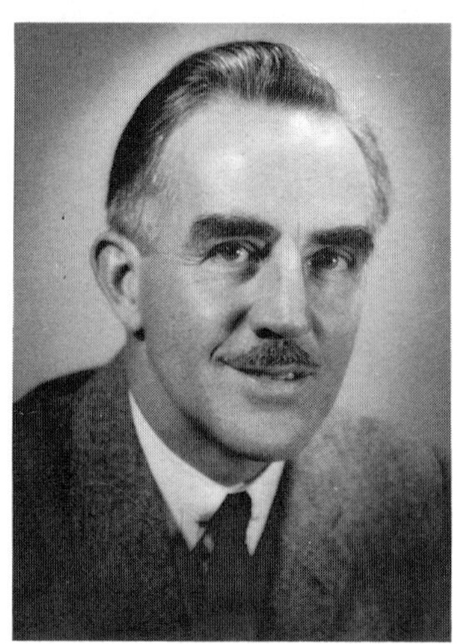

←
1968
Charles H. M. Williams

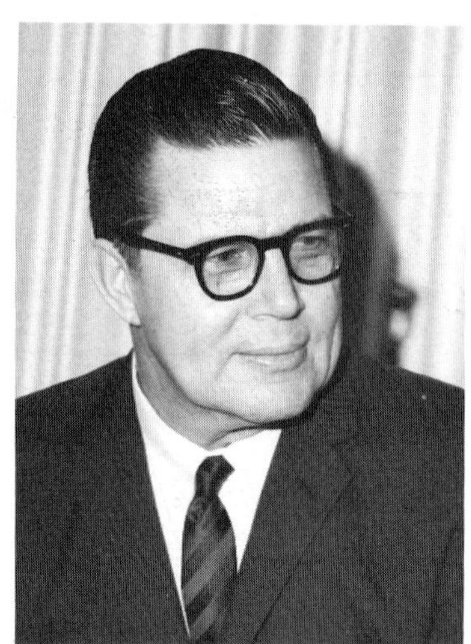

→
1969
Frank T. Scott

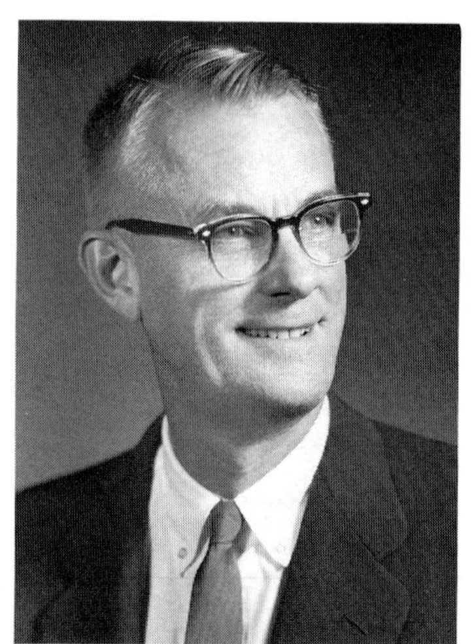

←
1970
Perry A. Ratcliff

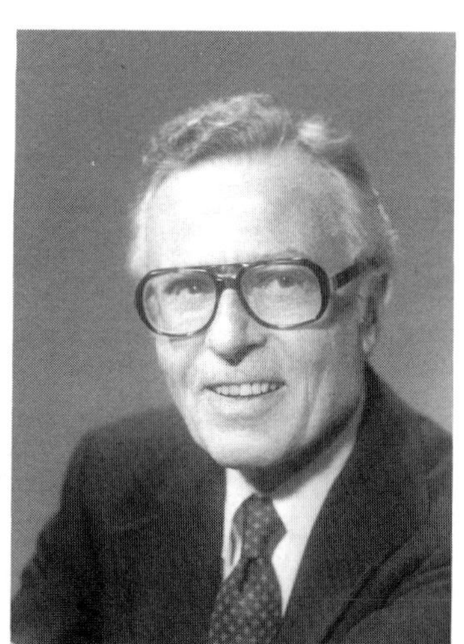

→
1971
Robert Gottsegen

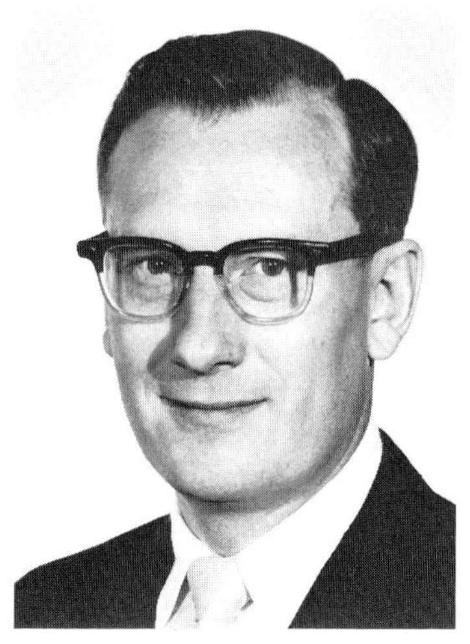

←

1972
Erwin M. Schaffer

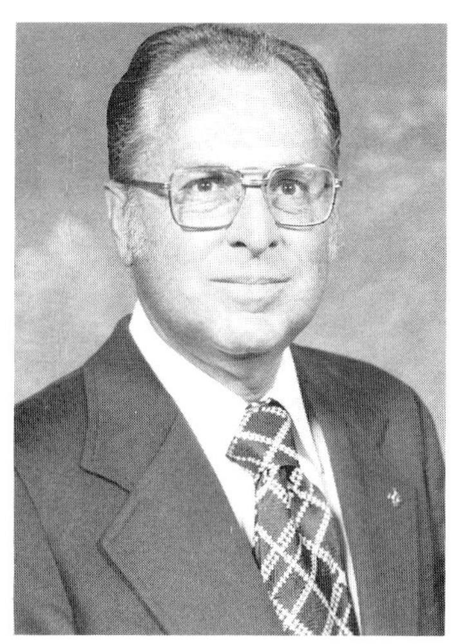

→

1973
Claude L. Nabers

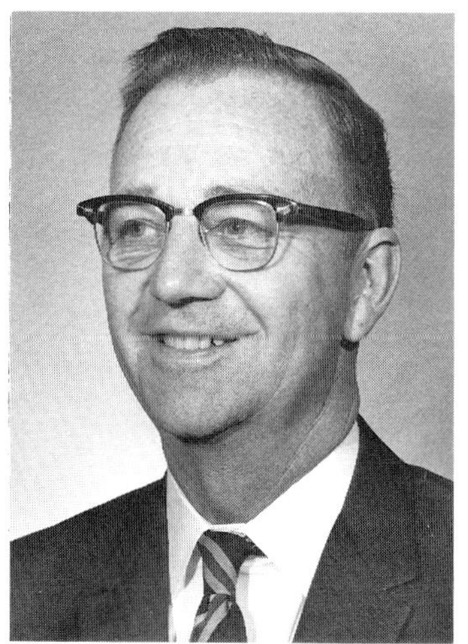

←

1974
Henry M. Swenson

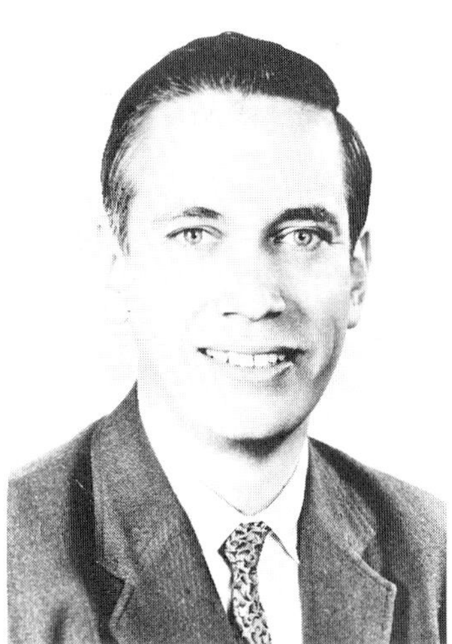

→

1975
Richard E. Stallard

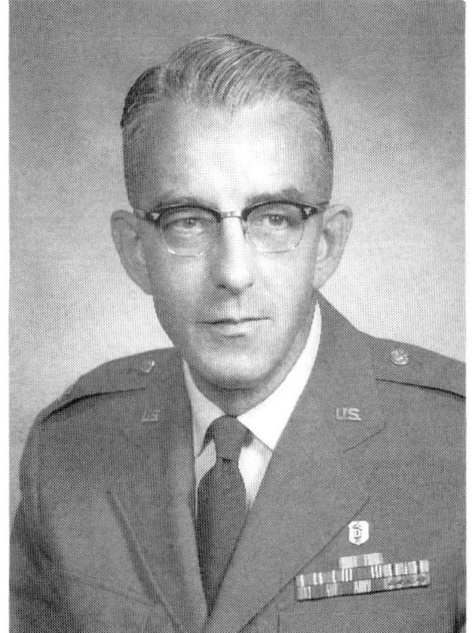

←

1976
Timothy J. O'Leary

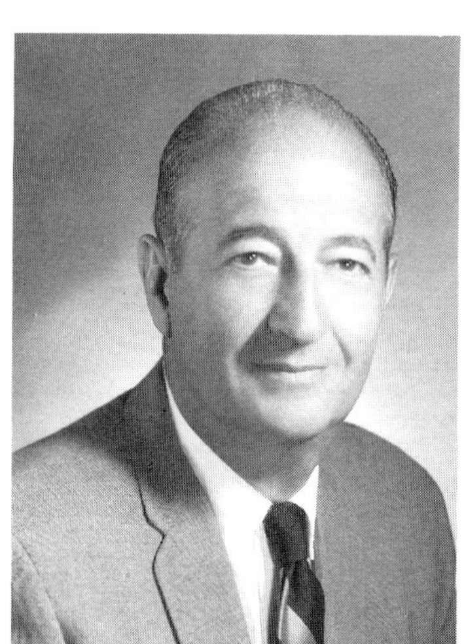

→

1977
Marvin M. Sugerman

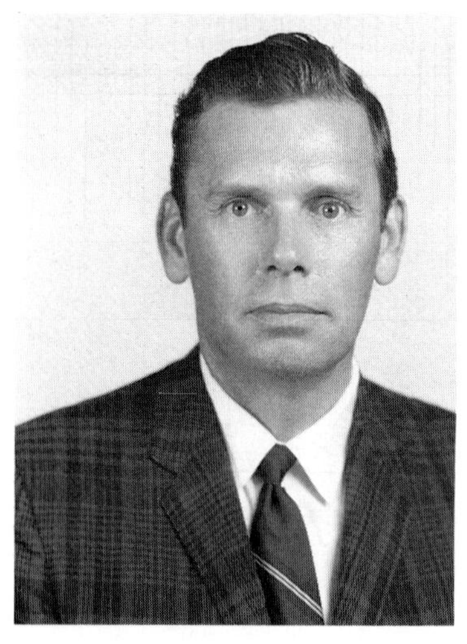

←

1978
James Y. O'Bannon, Jr.

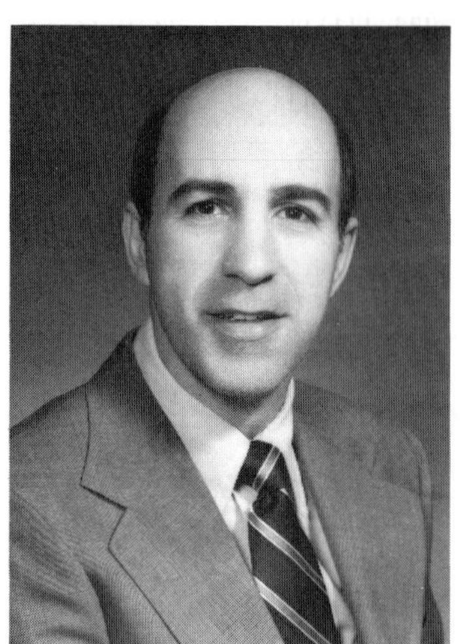

→

1979
Harry Staffileno

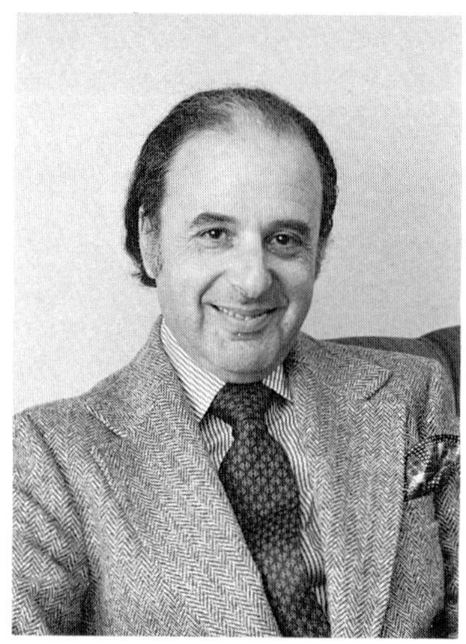

←

1980
S. Sigmund Stahl

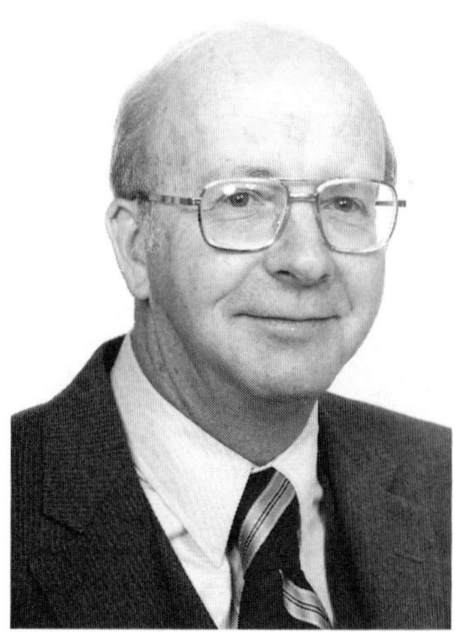

→

1981
Robert L. Reeves

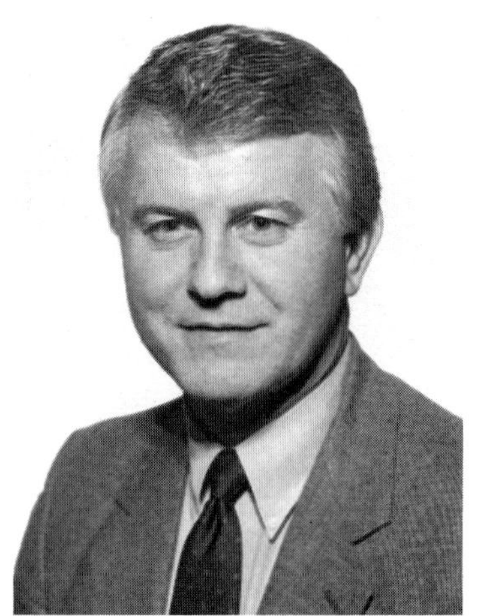

←

1982
James A. Tobias

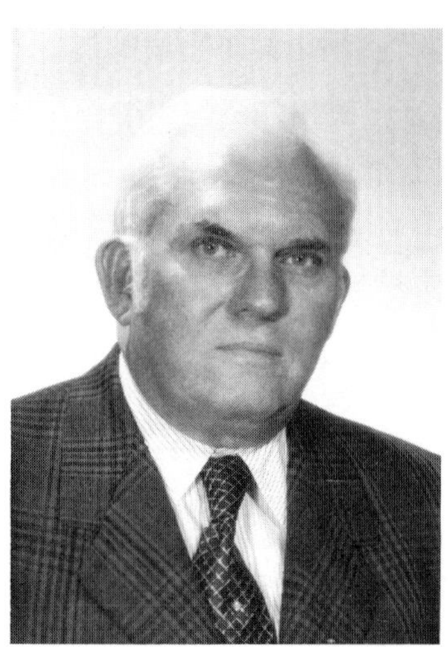

→

1983
Charles W. Finley

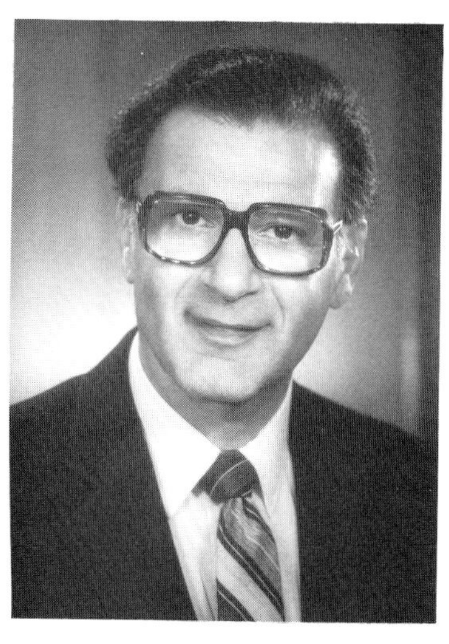

←
1984
Erwin P. Barrington

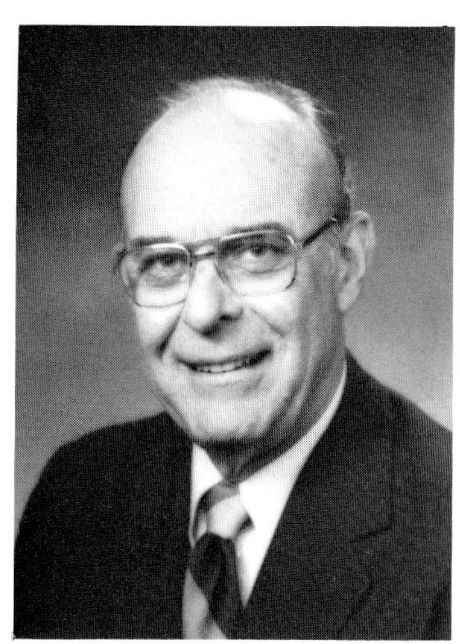

→
1985
Kenneth B. Langley

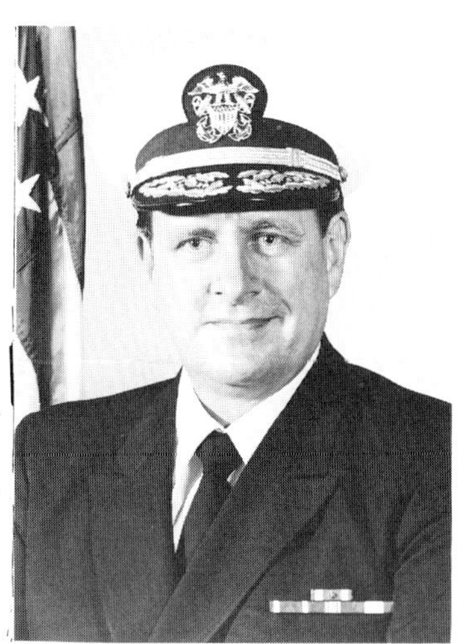

←
1986
Robert W. Koch

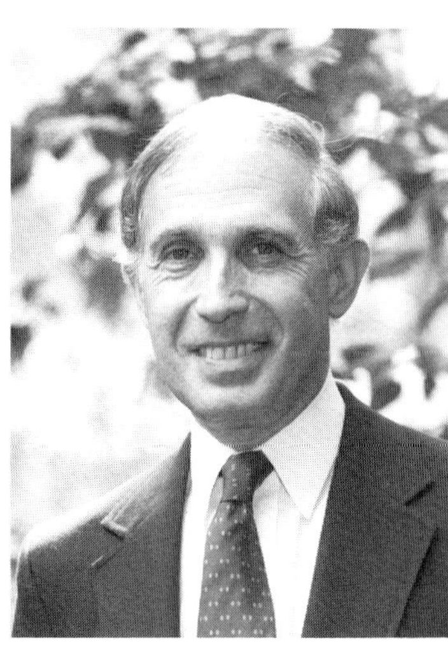

→
1987
Stephen F. Goodman

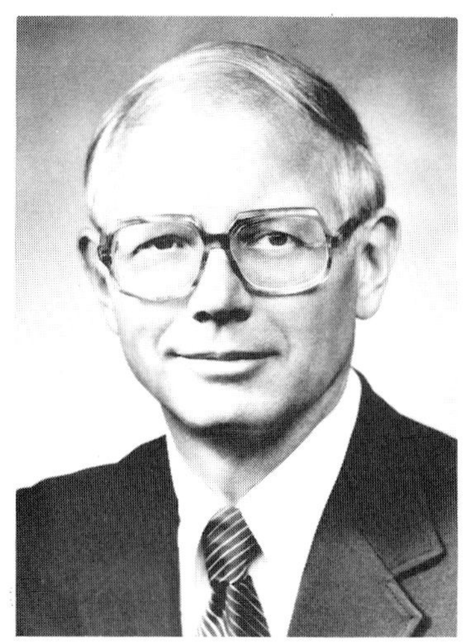

←
1988
Robert G. Schallhorn

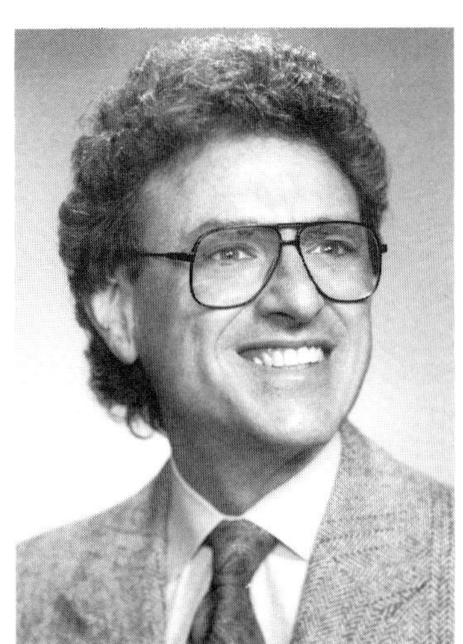

→
1989
Myron Nevins

Presidents of the
American Society of Periodontists

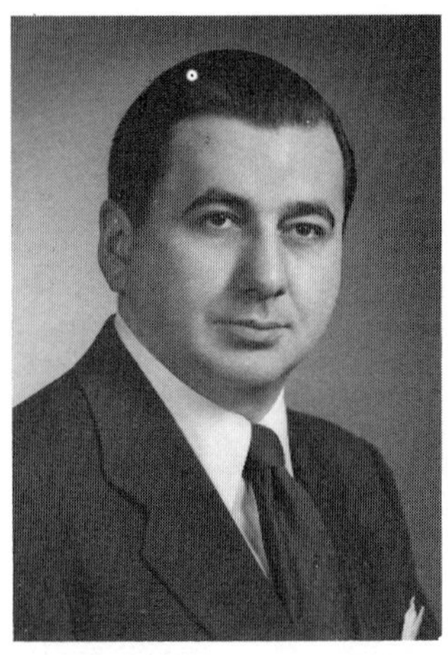

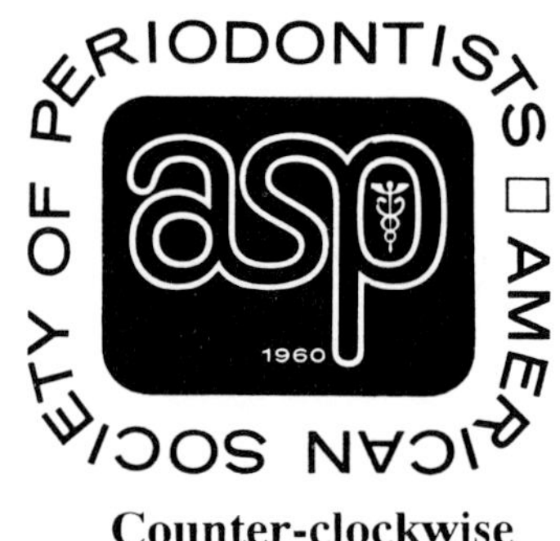

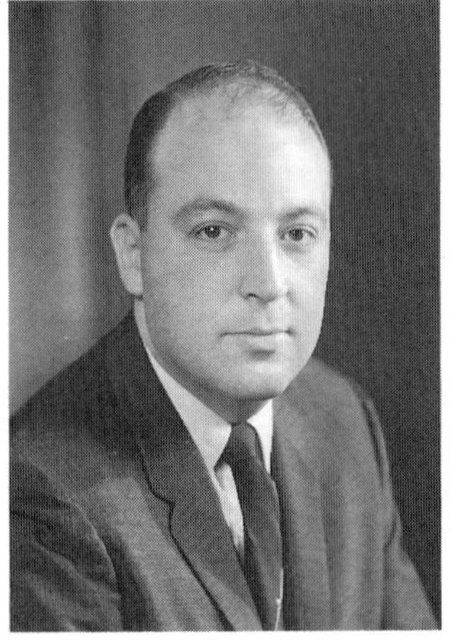

Counter-clockwise from upper left

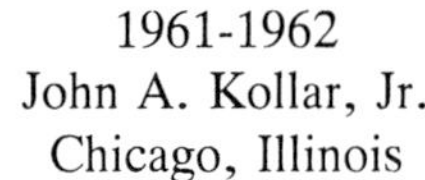

1961-1962
John A. Kollar, Jr.
Chicago, Illinois

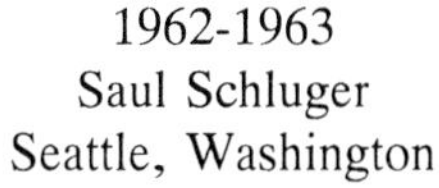

1962-1963
Saul Schluger
Seattle, Washington

1963-1964
Henry M. Goldman
Boston, Massachusetts

1964-1965
John F. Prichard
Fort Worth, Texas

1965
William H. Hiatt
Denver, Colorado

1966-1967
D. Walter Cohen
Philadelphia, Pennsylvania

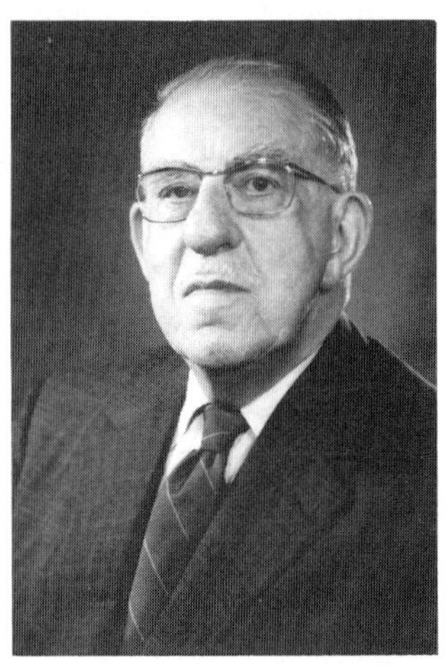

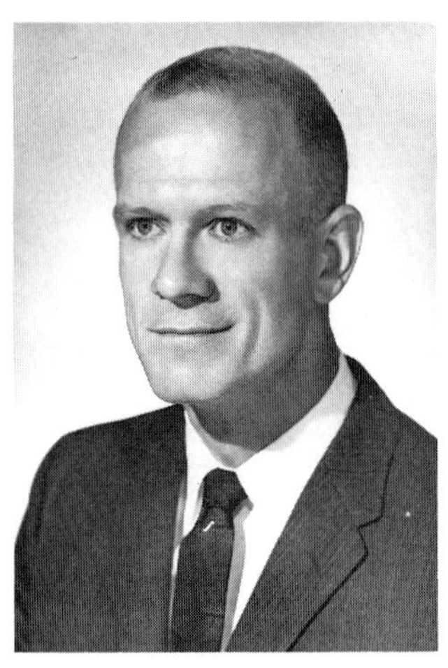

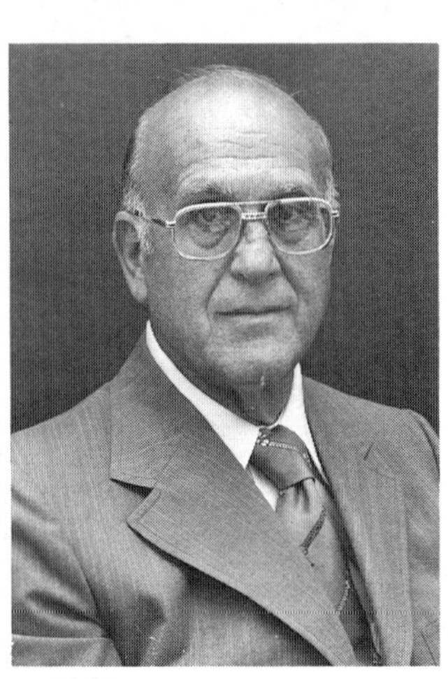

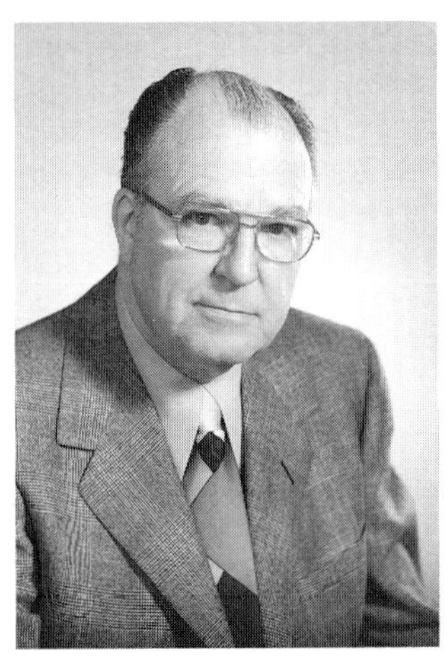

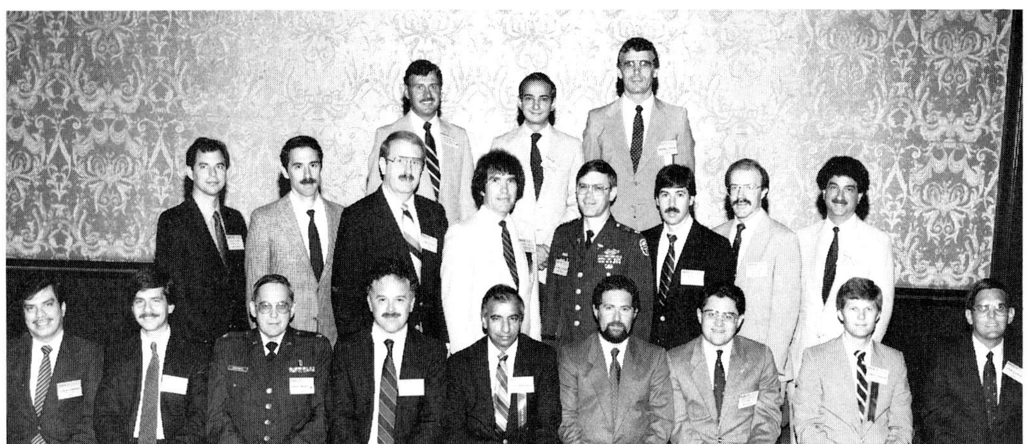

Two of the more recent "graduating" classes of the American Board of Periodontology: above, 1984 and below, 1987.

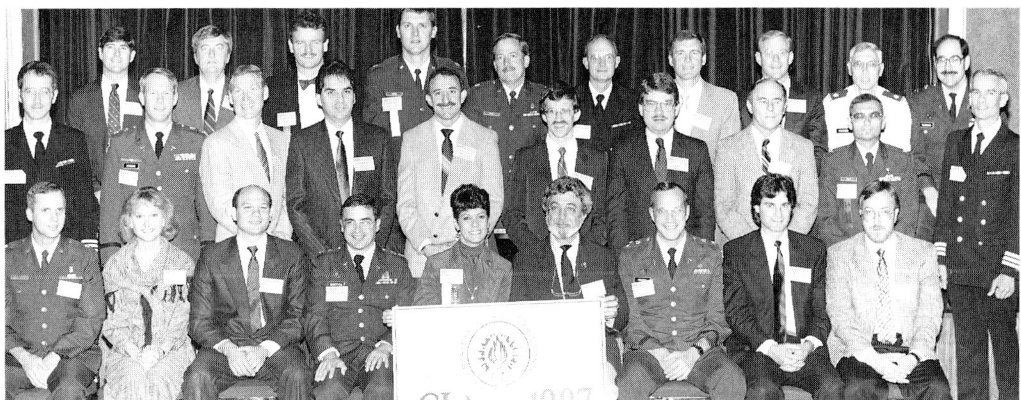

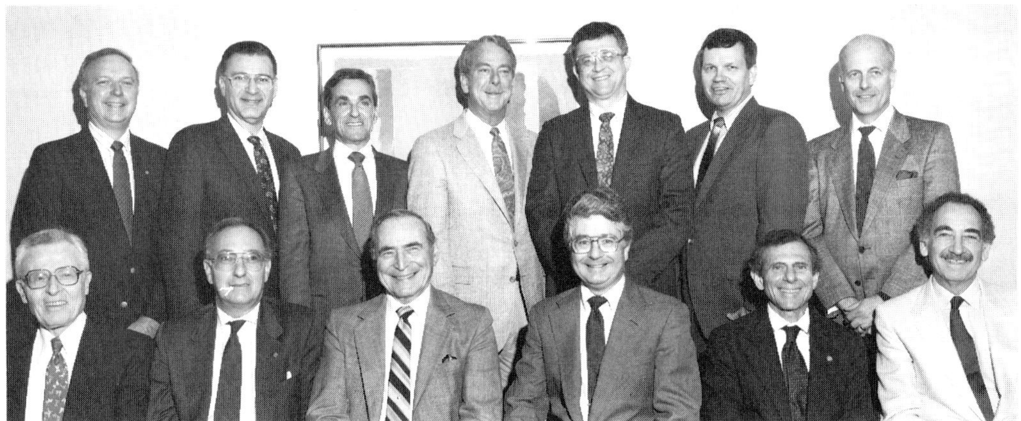

The American Board of Periodontology and 1989 examiners. First row, left to right: Robert Gottsegen, William Becker (1989 Vice Chairman), Abram Chasens, Philip Hoag (1989 Chairman), Walter Donnenfeld, and Anthony Gargiulo; second row, Gerald Bowers (Executive Secretary/Treasurer), Erwin Barrington, Daniel Grant, Jack Caton, James Mellonig, Ray Yukna, and Dan Loughlin.

Honors and Awards

The individuals shown on these two pages are representative of all of the recipients who have been honored by the Academy. A description of each of the awards and a complete list of recipients can be found on pages 00 to 00.

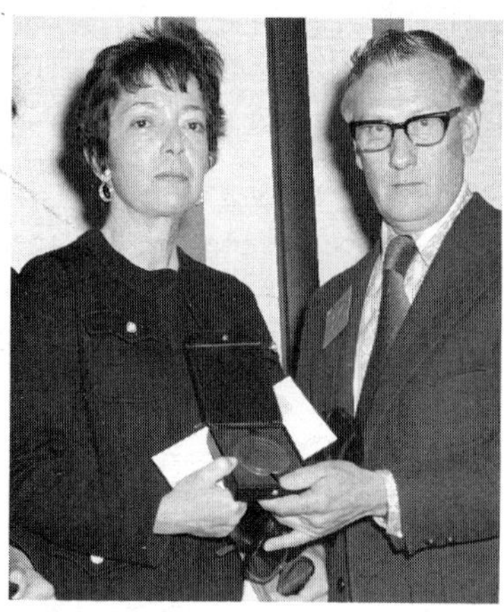

Violeta Arboleda accepts the 1972 **Gold Medal**, which was awarded posthumously to her husband Irving Glickman, from President Erwin M. Schaffer.

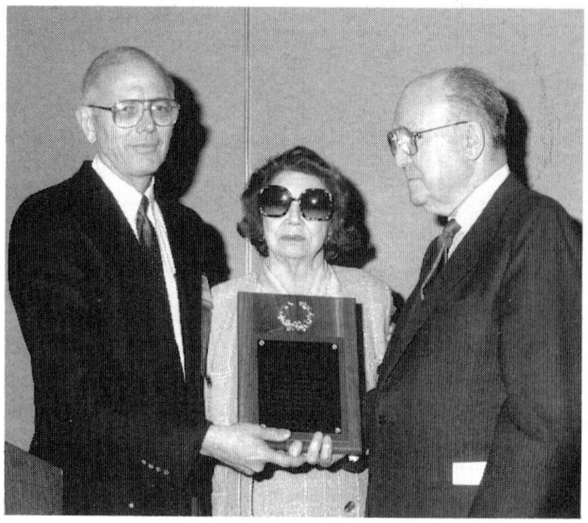

Dr. and Mrs. John Prichard accept congratulations from President Robert Schallhorn (left) at the 1988 Annual Meeting, where Dr. Prichard was presented with the **Master Clinician Award**.

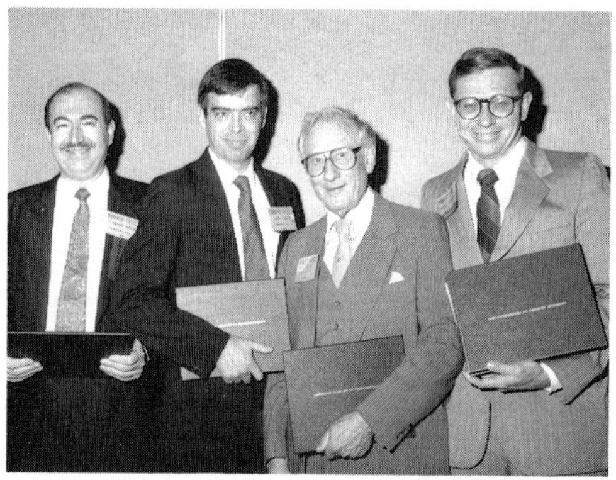

Four of the seven recipients of the 1988 **Clinical Research Award in Periodontology**, (from left) M. Bashar Bakdash, Larry F. Wolff, Erwin M. Schaffer, and Bruce L. Pihlstrom.

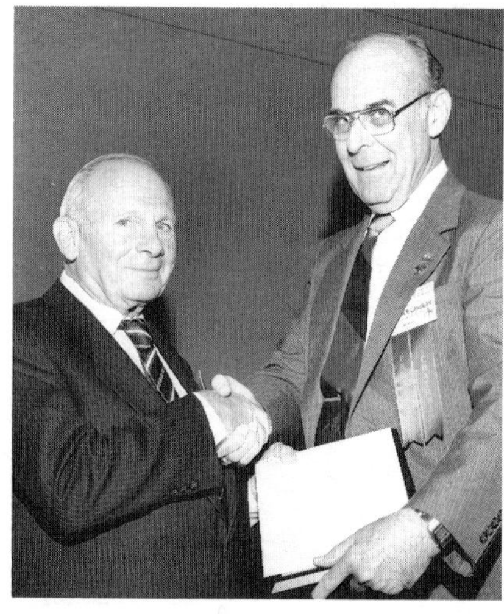

Helmut Zander (left) received the 1985 **Gies Award** from President Kenneth B. Langley.

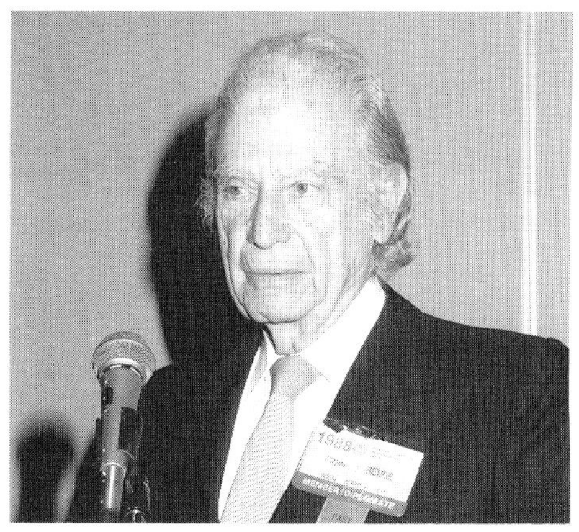

Frank Beube, 1988 **Presidential Award** recipient, delivers his acceptance speech.

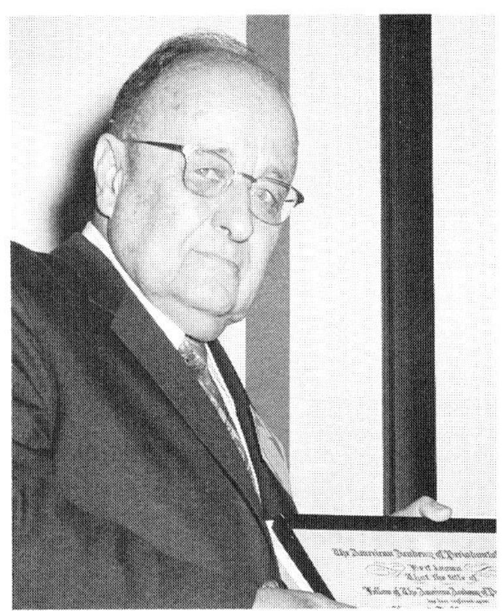

Howard Hartman, who served as the Academy's photographer for many years, was named a **Fellow** in 1972.

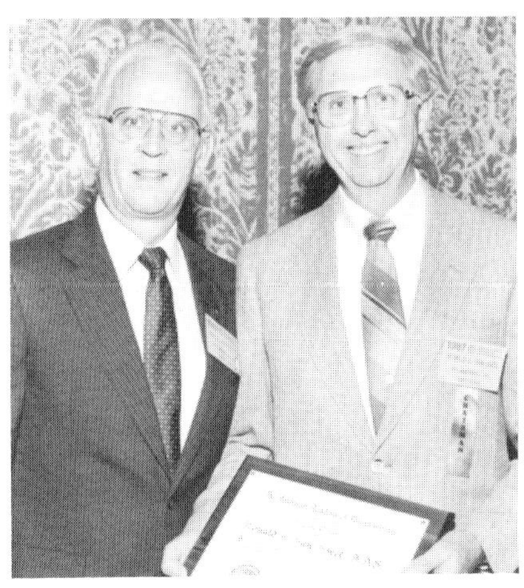

Ronald Van Swol (right) was escorted by Donald Van Scotter when he received his **Special Citation** in 1987.

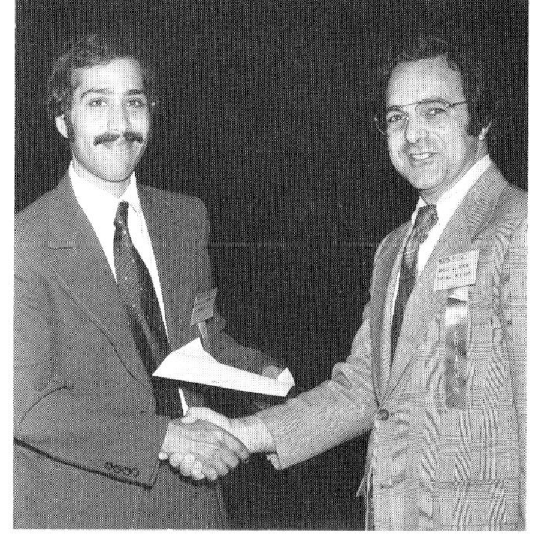

In 1975, the **Orban Prize** winner was Michael G. Newman (left) and the committee chairman was Robert J. Genco; today, they are, respectively, Secretary of the Academy and Editor of the *Journal of Periodontology*.

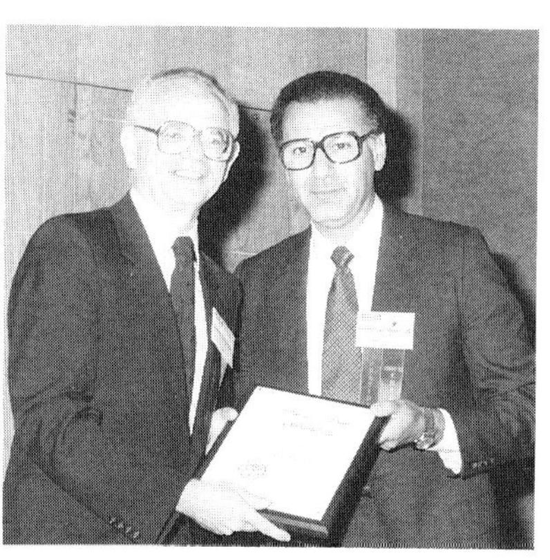

Sigmund Socransky received his **Honorary Membership** from President Erwin Barrington in 1984.

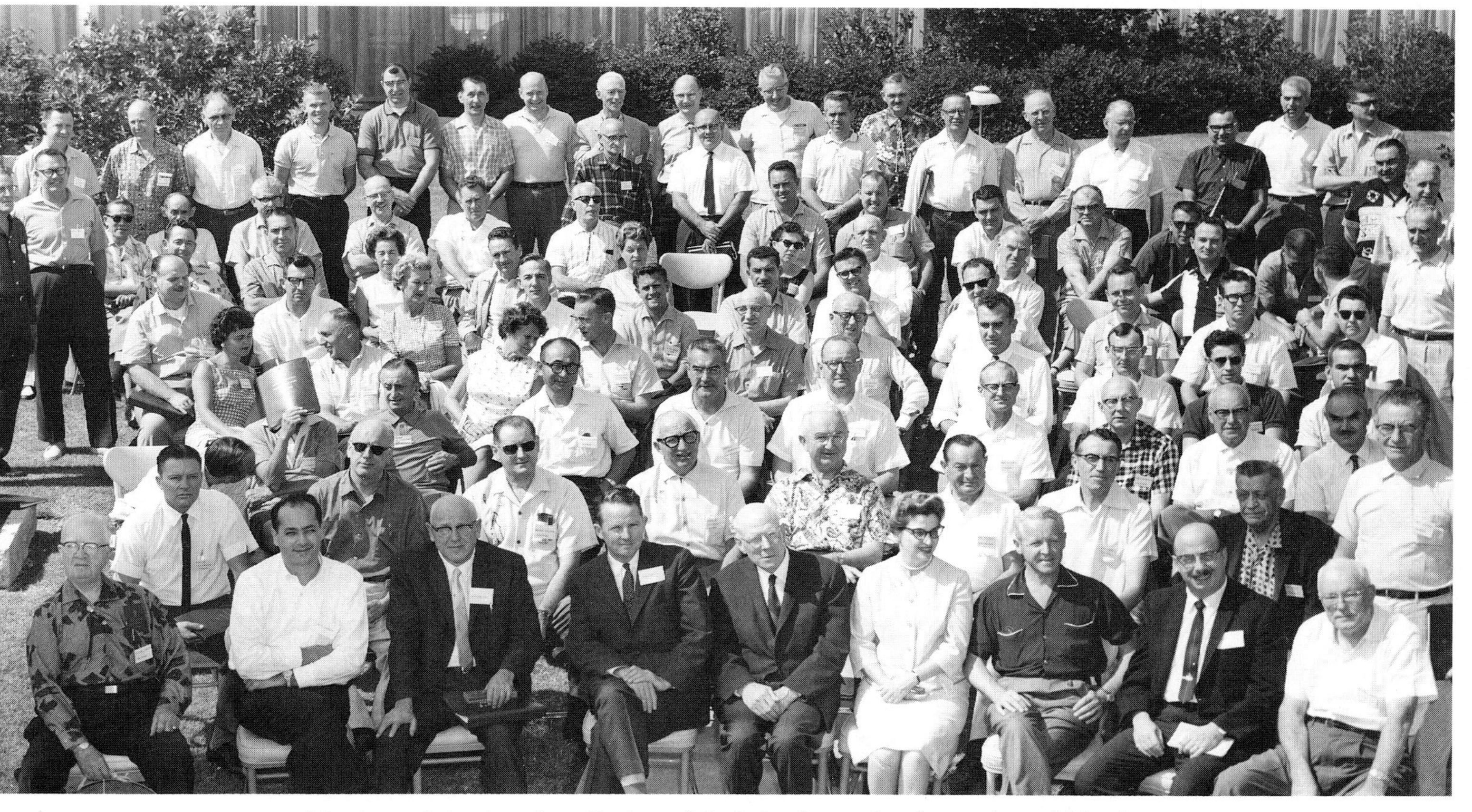

Members of the American Society of Periodontists gather for an Annual Meeting.

American Society of Periodontists

The photographs on these two pages highlight ASP activities.

(right) Sumter Arnim (on right) received the first Gold Medal, an award established by the Society, from ASP President D. Walter Cohen in 1967.

(below) Harold Schreiber, Luke Howlett, Jr., George Lawther, and Thomas E. Prosser at the Society Annual Meeting in Chicago.

(bottom) Another group setting at a Society Annual Meeting.

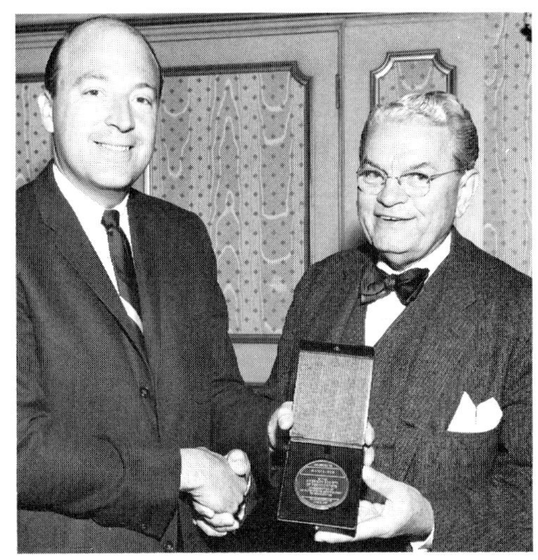

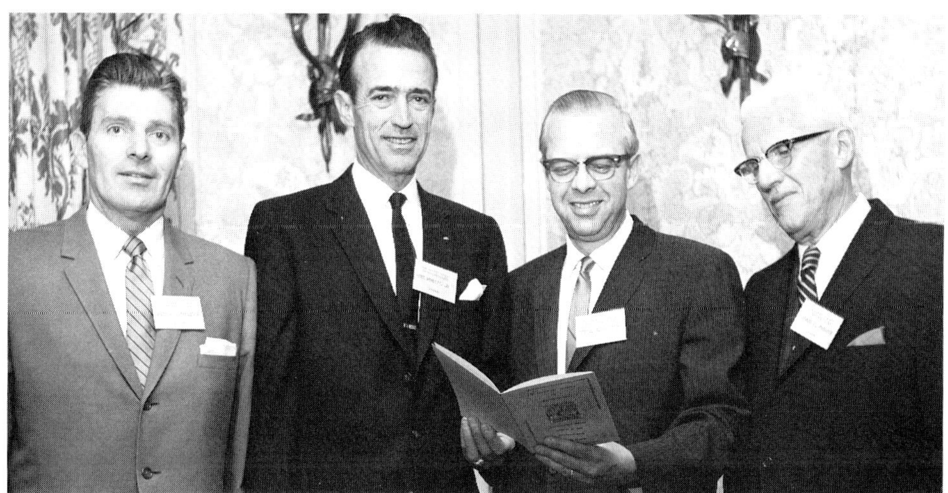

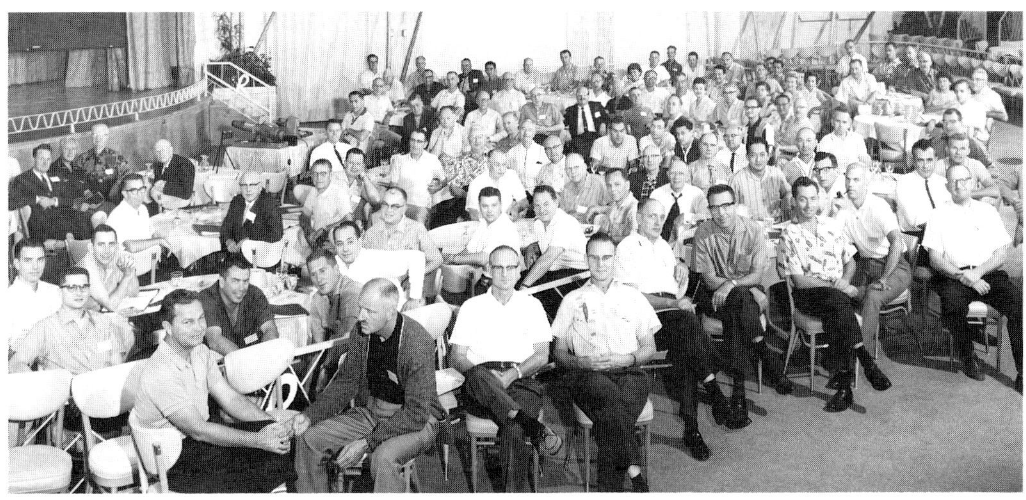

Annual Meeting Montage

The next six pages contain a selection of sights, scenes, and people primarily from the 1951 (Washington, DC) through the 1988 (San Diego, California) Annual Meetings of the Academy.

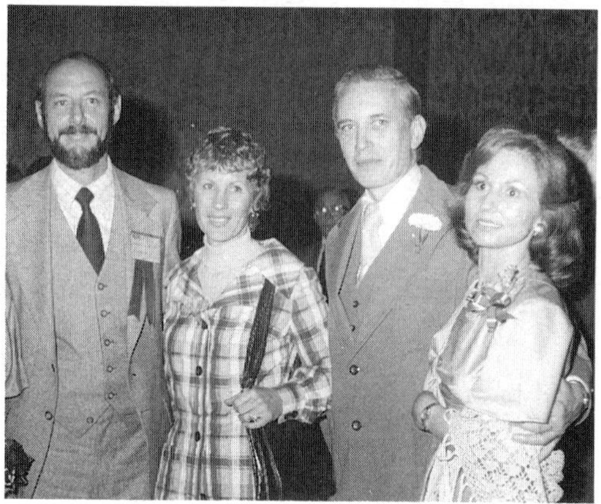

Dr. and Mrs. Richard Stallard (right) with Dr. and Mrs. Gil Oliver at the 1976 meeting.

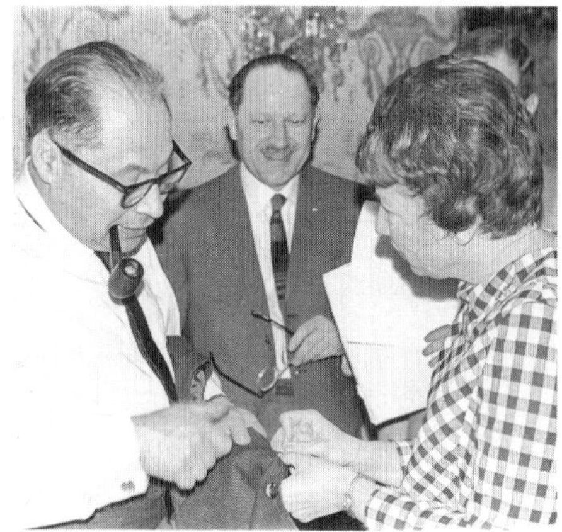

Marilyn Holmquist demonstrates one of her many talents as she sews on a button for Irving Glickman while Paul Baer waits his turn!

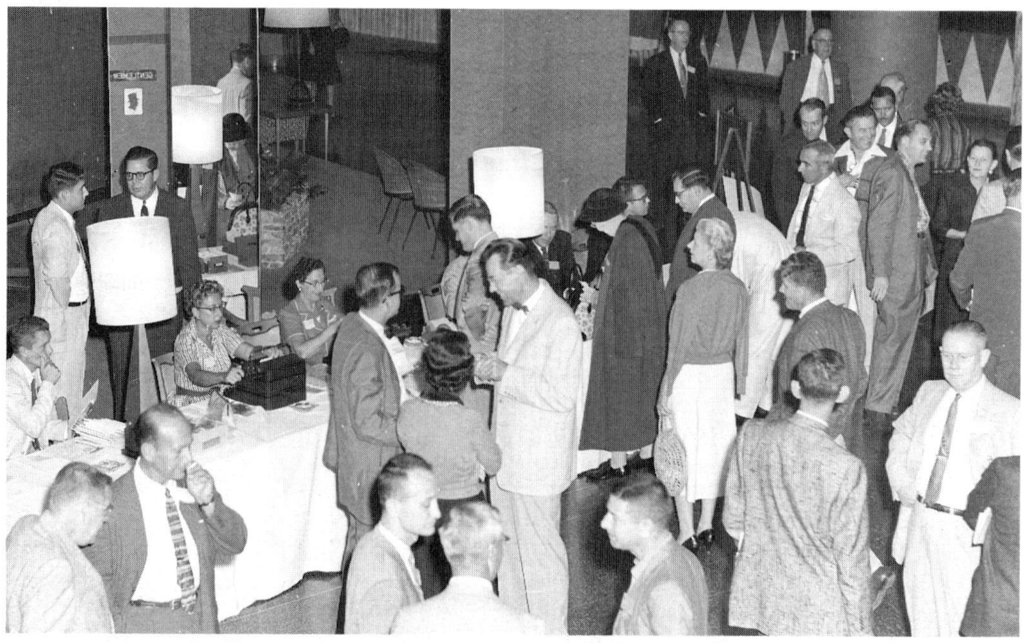

Registration as it was in the 1950s—when typewriters represented the latest in sophisticated office equipment.

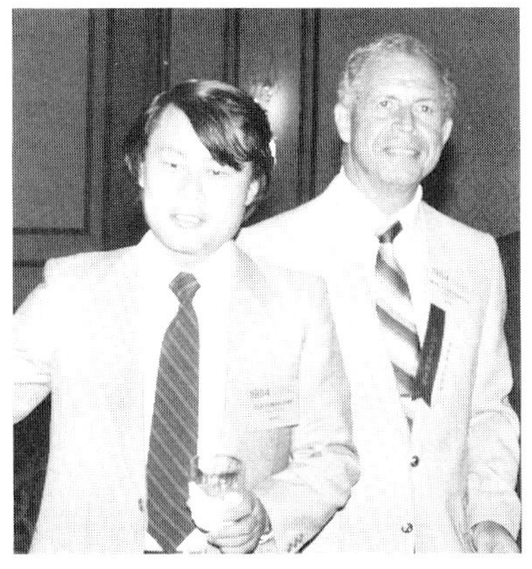

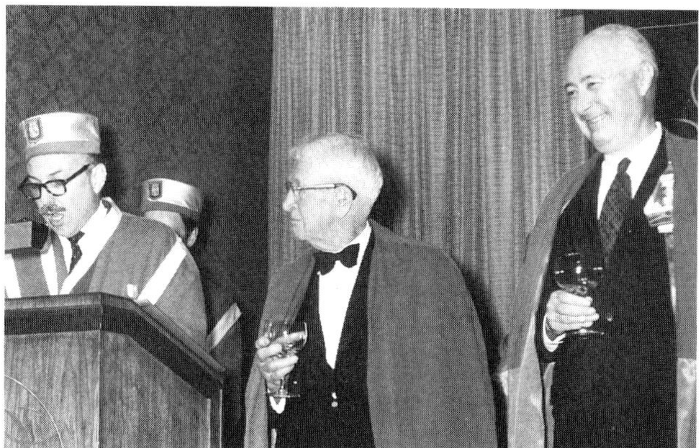

(above) Eiji Funakoshi and Max Listgarten at the 1984 Annual Meeting in New Orleans.

(above right) The 1970 Annual Meeting in Montreal included pagentry and fun. From left: Charles Tonneau, A.W. Ward and Sigurd Ramfjord, appear to have enjoyed the festivities.

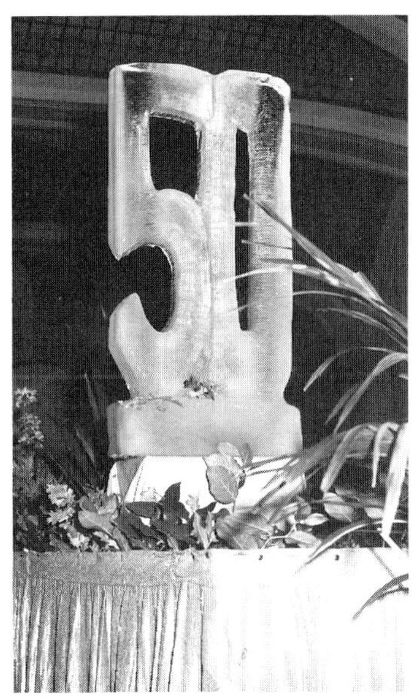

(right) The 50th anniversary celebration in 1964 (San Francisco) included this ice sculpture.

(below right) Hunter Allen and Mildred Dickerson confer.

(below) Current and former Editors of the *Journal of Periodontology* at the 1988 Annual Meeting in San Diego. From left, Robert J. Genco, Timothy J. O'Leary, William C. Hurt, and Maynard K. Hine.

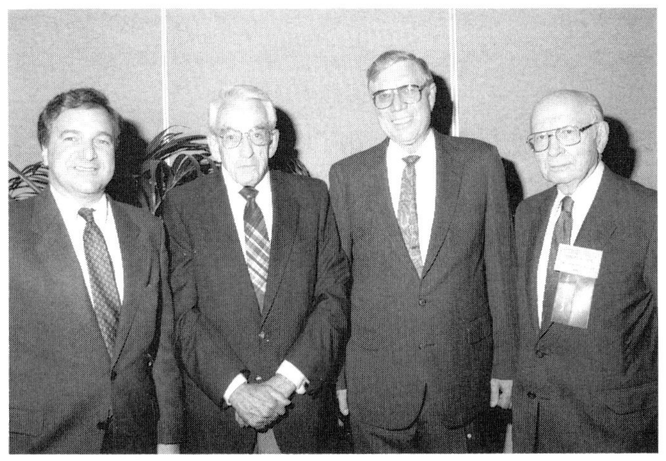

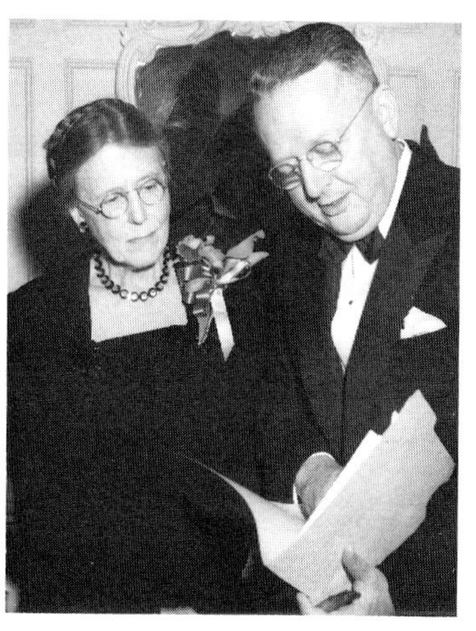

In the 1950s, members provided the entertainment as well as the scientific program. This fine orchestra performed at the 1951 Annual meeting in Washington, DC.

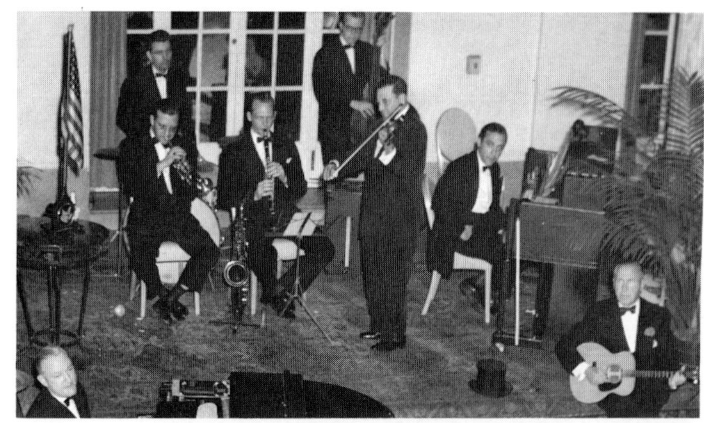

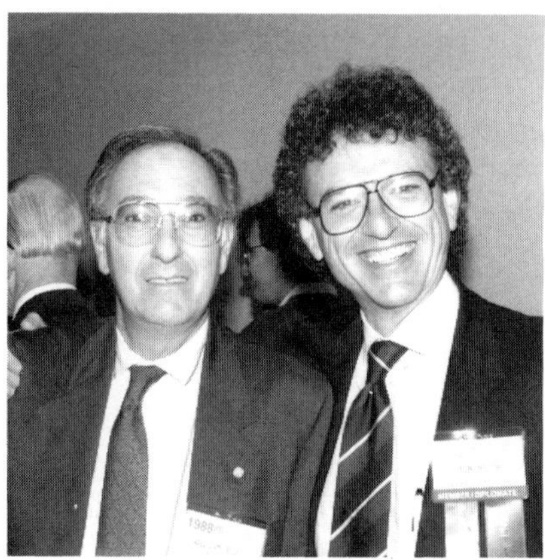

1989 Vice President William Becker (left) and 1989 President Myron Nevins relax at the 1988 meeting in San Diego.

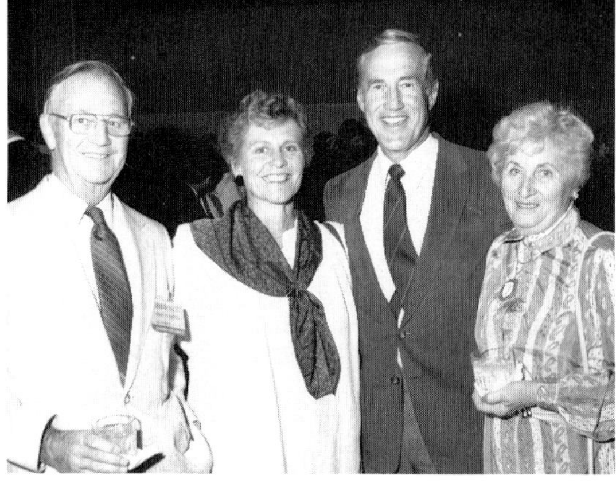

Dr. and Mrs. Henry Swenson enjoy a relaxing moment with Dr. and Mrs. Dick Oliver.

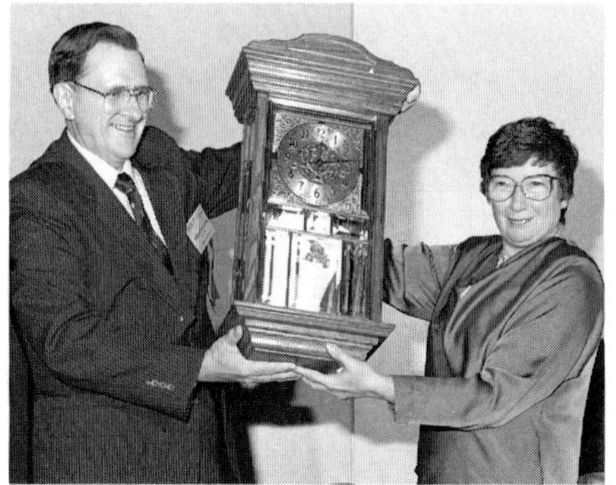

Assisted by Robert Koch, retiring Executive Director Marilyn Holmquist proudly displays one of the many gifts she received from a grateful Academy membership (Cleveland, 1986).

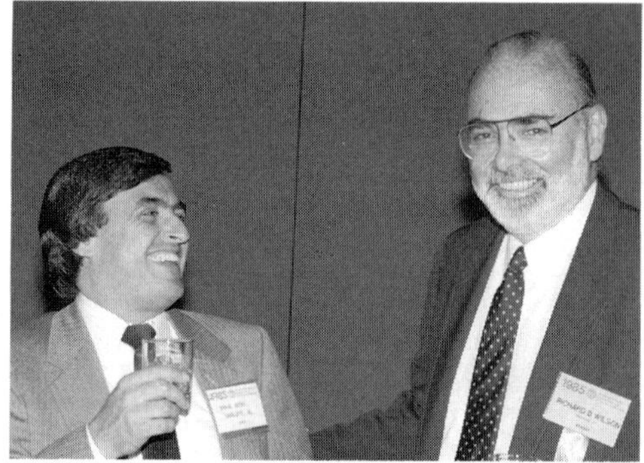

Robert Rucho (left) in conversation with Richard Wilson, Associate Member Representative on the Executive Council (San Francisco, 1985).

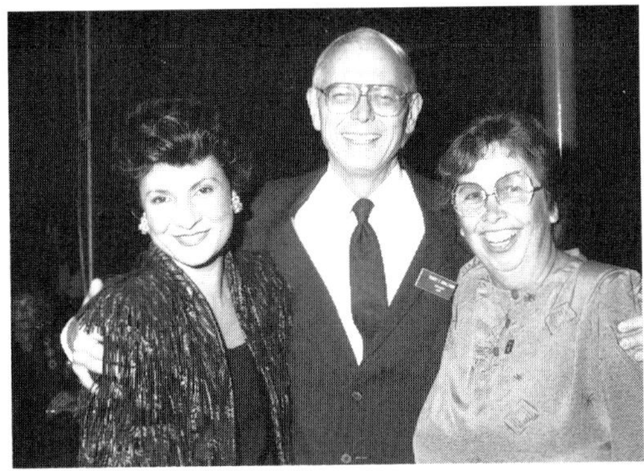

1988 President Robert G. Schallhorn relaxes with Mrs. Schallhorn (right) and Executive Director Alice DeForest at the 1988 President's Party (San Diego).

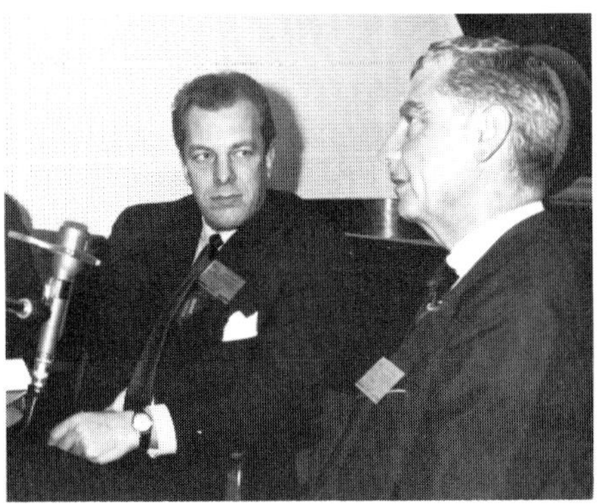

Harald Löe and Frank Beube at a recording studio during the 1964 meeting in San Francisco.

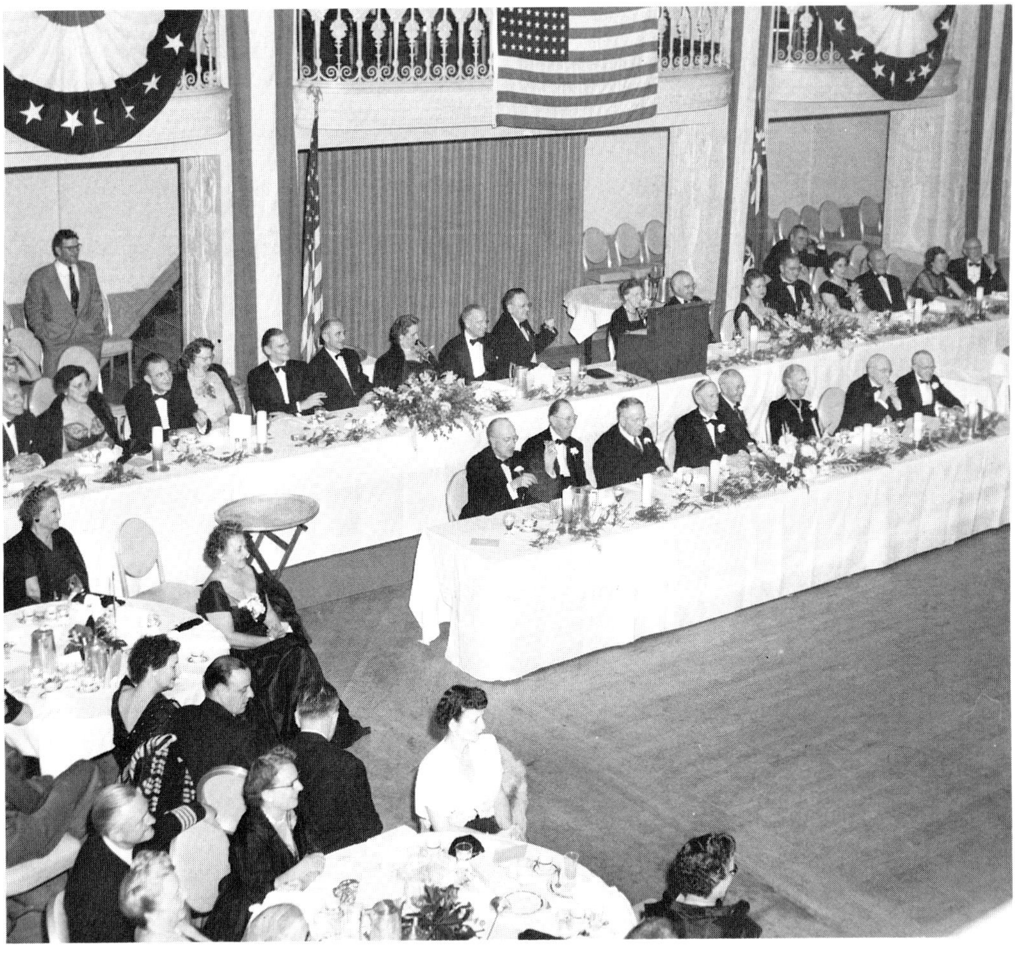

The 1951 Annual Meeting in Washington, DC included a formal black tie banquet.

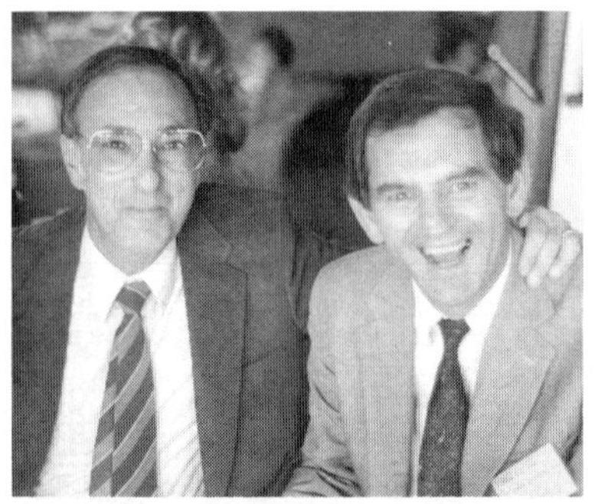

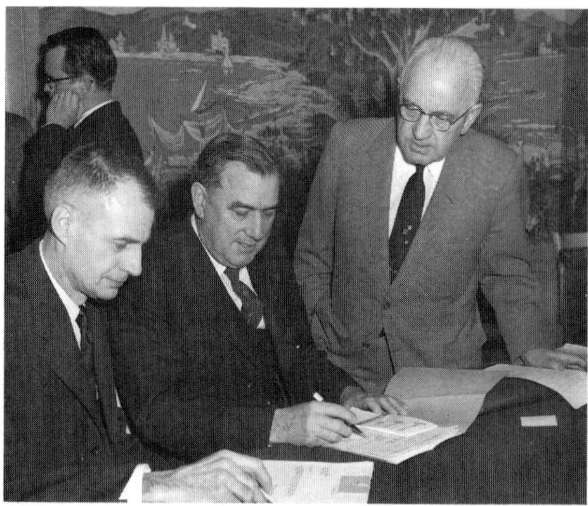

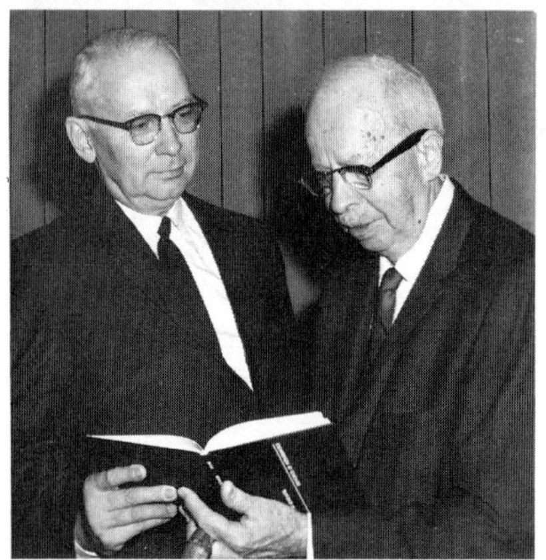

Clockwise, from upper left.

1989 Vice President William Becker and President Elect J. Gary Maynard, Jr. share an amusing moment in Anaheim (1982).

Three busy and intent officers (from left) Delbert Nachazel, Stanley C. Baker and Clarke Chamberlain confer.

On the left, 1987 President and Mrs. Stephen F. Goodman and on the right, Dr. and Mrs. Sebastian Ciancio find time to smile in Denver.

R. Earl Robinson and Walter T. McFall, Jr. in conversation during the 1985 Annual Meeting in San Francisco.

Herman (left) and Jack Corn; one of several father and son memberships found in the Academy (1987).

1964 President Maynard K. Hine with the Academy's third President, John Oppie McCall, during the 50th Anniversary celebration in San Francisco.

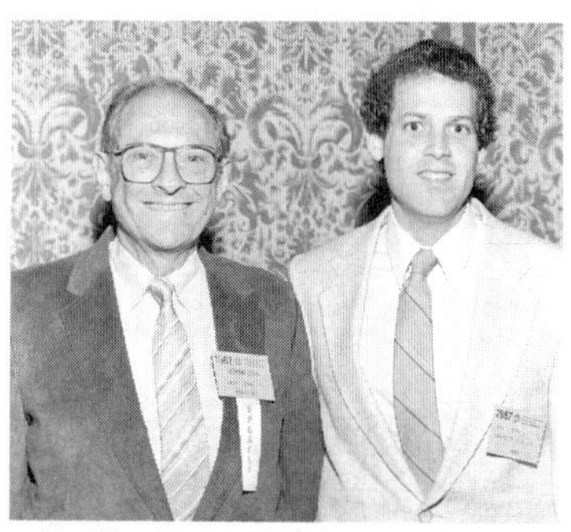

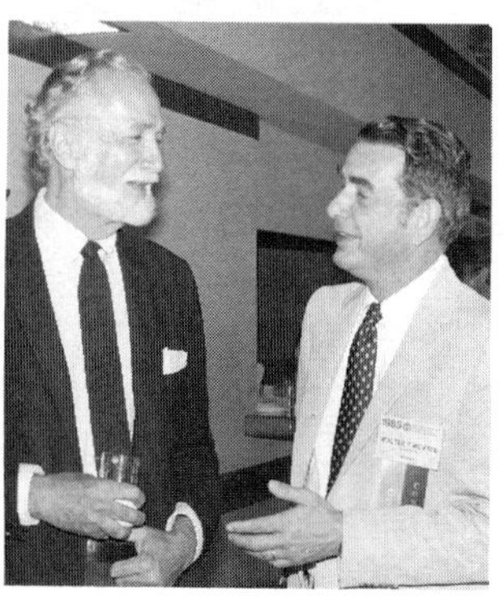

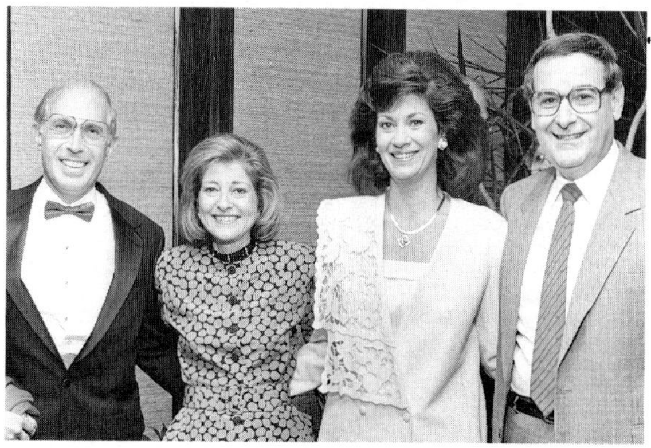

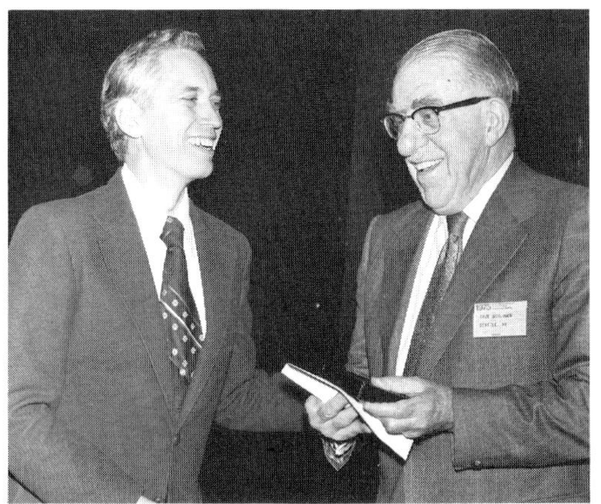

Then AAP president Richard Stallard and former ASP president Saul Schluger share a laugh at the 1975 Annual Meeting in Minneapolis.

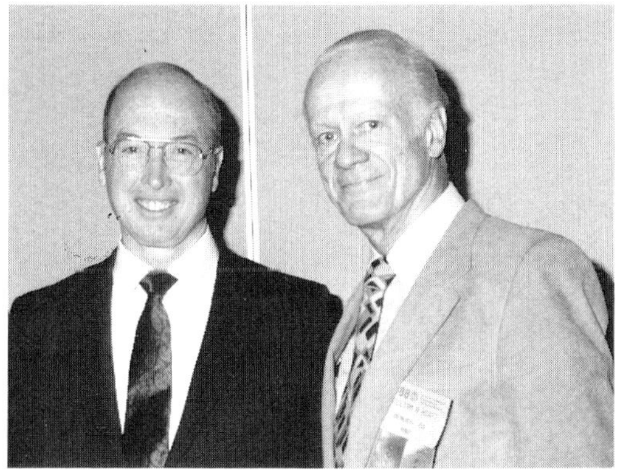

Two of Colorado's favorite sons, H. Dalton Conner (left) and William Hiatt (right), at the 1988 Annual Meeting in San Diego.

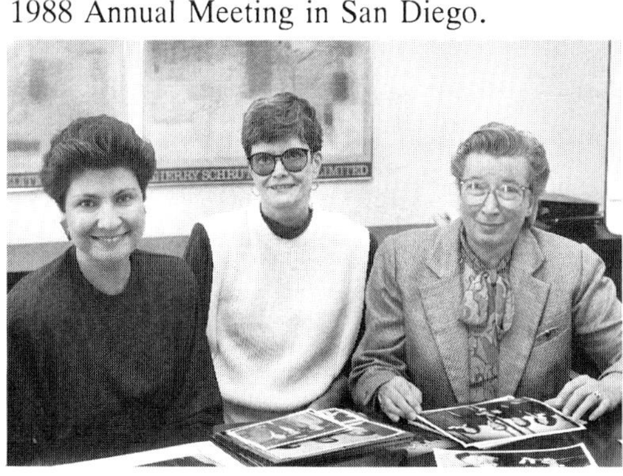

AAP Executive Director Alice DeForest (left) and former Executive Director Marilyn Holmquist (right) worked with AAP staff member Rita Shafer (center) to select photographs for the *History*.

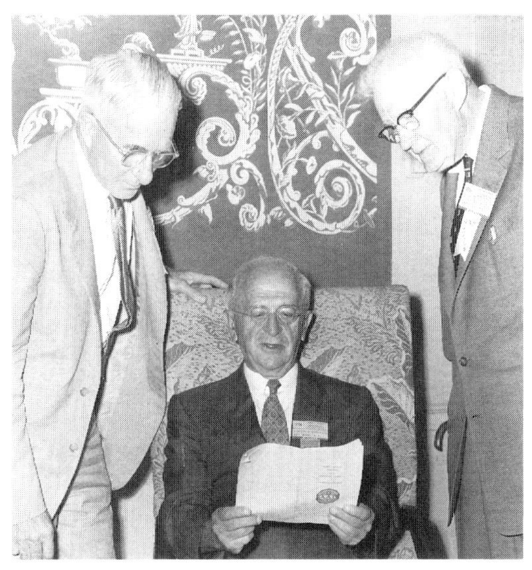

Three former presidents (from left) Harold J. Leonard (1932), Isador Hirschfeld (1941), and Edgar D. Coolidge (1947) examine the 1956 Annual meeting program. (Atlantic City)

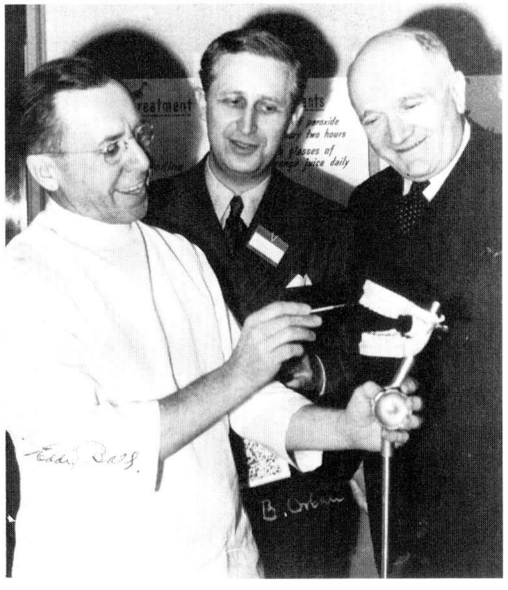

Edward Ball (left) gives an illustrated lecture to Balint Orban and Bernhard Gottlieb.

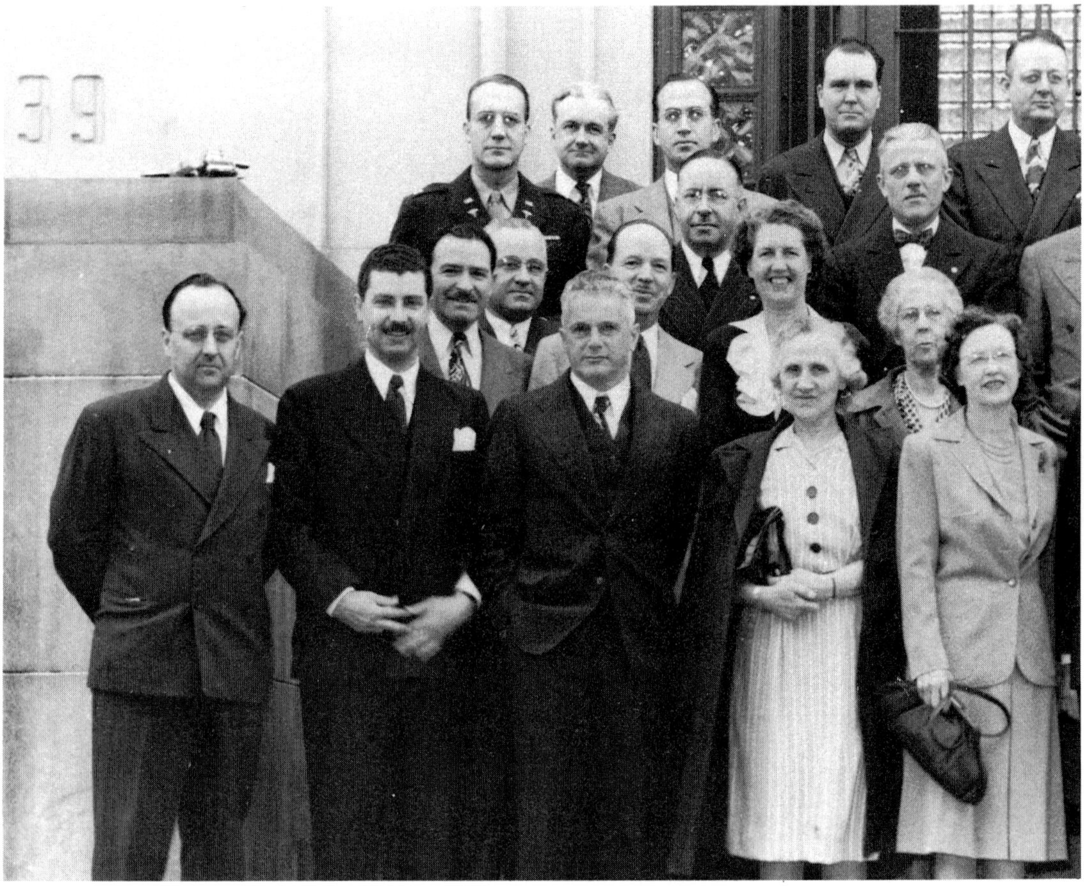

1. not identified
2. not identified
3. Henry Goldman
4. John Prichard
5. Hunter Allen
6. Howard Hartman
7. Frank Beube
8. Bernard S. Chaikin

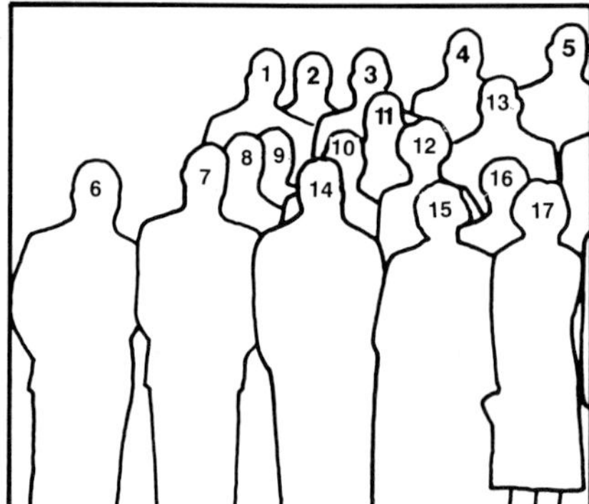

9. Clarke Chamberlain
10. not identified
11. Charles H. Buck
12. Dorothy Hard Bunting
13. not identified
14. Myer Wolfsohn
15. Grace Rogers Spalding
16. Cecilia Rich
17. Edith Davis

This photograph (above and above right) was taken at the University of Michigan in Ann Arbor during the early to mid 1940s. The author is indebted to members of the Academy who assisted in identifying these individuals; unfortunately, it was not possible to determine the identity of all those shown.

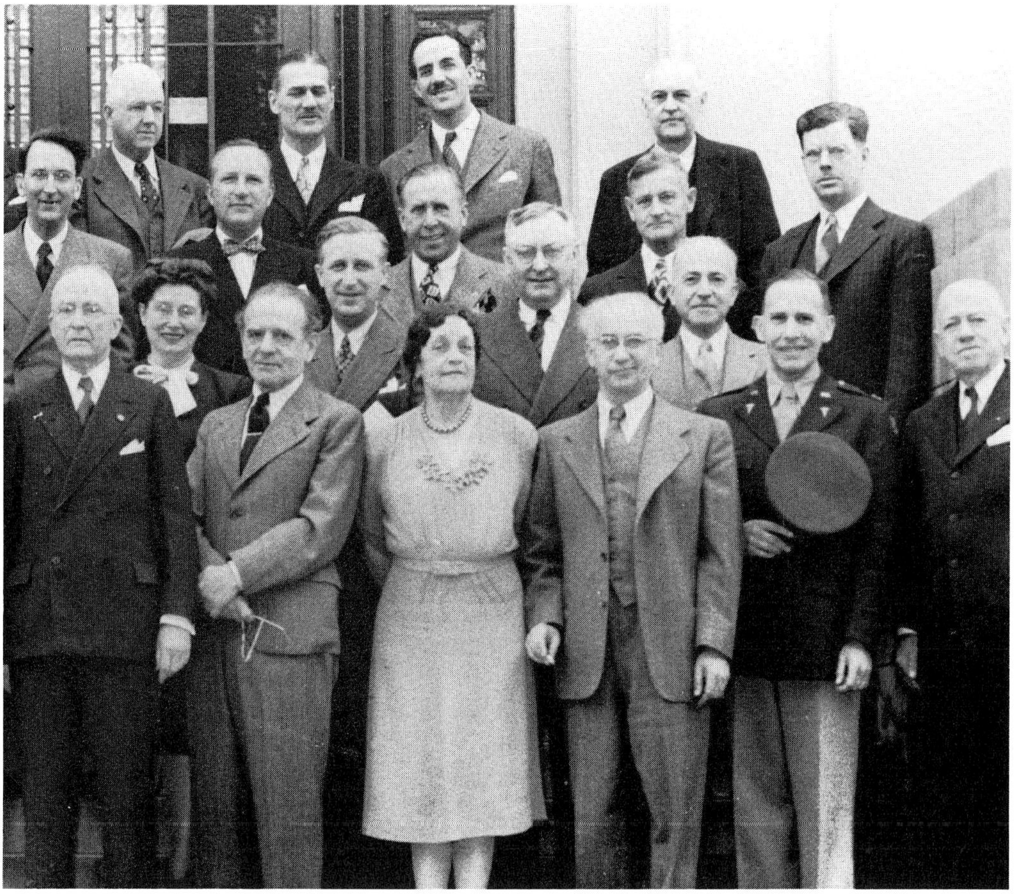

1. not identified
2. Frank Adams
3. Harold Ray
4. Raymond Johnson
5. Charles Williams
6. not identified
7. not identified
8. Arthur Merritt
9. Willa Yeretsky

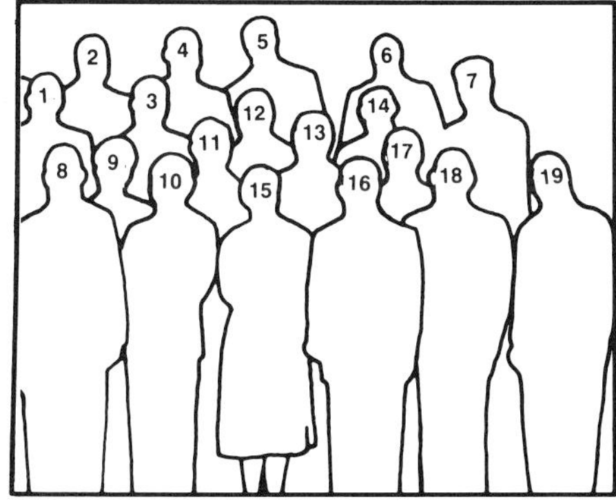

10. Harry Sicher
11. Balint Orban
12. Edward Ball
13. Sam Parks
14. not identified
15. not identified
16. Joseph Peter Weinman
17. Leon Wiesstien
18. not identified
19. not identified